Imene BOUJELBENE

Syndromic agenesis of the corpus callosum

Imene BOUJELBENE

Syndromic agenesis of the corpus callosum

Epidemiological, clinical and genetic study

ScienciaScripts

Imprint

Cover image: www.ingimage.com

This book is a translation from the original published under ISBN 978-620-6-72371-4.

Publisher:
Sciencia Scripts
is a trademark of
Dodo Books Indian Ocean Ltd. and OmniScriptum S.R.L publishing group

120 High Road, East Finchley, London, N2 9ED, United Kingdom
Str. Armeneasca 28/1, office 1, Chisinau MD-2012, Republic of Moldova, Europe
Printed at: see last page
ISBN: 978-620-8-14535-4

PLAN

Introduction

INTRODUCTION

The corpus callosum (CC) is the main interhemispheric commissure, comprising around 2 to 3% of all cortical fibres [Appendix 1: Anatomy of the corpus callosum]. (1). It transfers sensory, motor and cognitive information between the two cerebral hemispheres and plays a fundamental role in executive functions, social interaction and language. (2).

Agenesis of the corpus callosum (ACC) corresponds to a complete or partial absence of formation of the CC. It is the most common cerebral malformation in newborns (3,4). It is diagnosed mainly by cerebral MRI, which can also be used to identify any associated cerebral malformations.

In 51% of cases, ACC is associated with other malformations (cerebral or extra-cerebral anomalies). These syndromic forms often have an unfavourable cognitive prognosis compared with isolated forms, in which 70% of children have normal intellectual development (1,5). Both isolated and syndromic ACCs are highly heterogeneous from a genetic point of view, and are part of known syndromes in around a third of cases.

The objectives of this work were to :

1) To determine the clinical and epidemiological characteristics of a series of patients with syndromic agenesis of the corpus callosum.

2) To emphasise the importance of the clinical examination in the etiological orientation of syndromic agenesis of the corpus callosum

Patients & Methods

PATIENTS AND METHODS

1. TYPE OF STUDY

We conducted a single-centre, descriptive, retrospective study of a cohort of patients with agenesis of the corpus callosum.

2. STUDY POPULATION

2.1. Inclusion criteria

We included in this study all patients with complete (ACCc) or partial (ACCp) agenesis of the corpus callosum diagnosed postnatally by brain MRI.

2.2 Criteria for non-inclusion

The criteria for non-inclusion in our study were as follows:

- ACC diagnosed prenatally with no postnatal follow-up.
- ACC diagnosed only by a brain scan.
- ACC considered to be secondary either to a principal malformation (such as neural tube defects) or to a major disorder of the diverticulation of the cerebral vesicle (such as porencephaly).
- Presence of signs of foetal distress on brain MRI.
- Hypoplasia of the corpus callosum: a thinner corpus callosum but with a normal anterior-posterior extent.

3. DATA COLLECTION

3.1 Data sources

Data were collected from the handwritten medical records of the Congenital and Hereditary Diseases Department at Charles Nicolle Hospital in Tunis.

3.2. Data collected

We drew up a form to record the patient's history, physical examination and specialist or paraclinical examinations [Appendix 2]. The data collected for each of our patients were as follows:

3.2.1. Patient identity

We noted the file number, surname, first name, sex and age at the first and last consultations.

3.2.2. Family history

We noted consanguinity, parents' geographical origins, family history of corpus callosum malformation and/or other neurological history.

3.2.3. Monitoring pregnancy and childbirth

We specified the mother's age at conception, the course of the pregnancy, whether or not she had taken any toxic substances or medication during the pregnancy, whether or not there were any prenatal signs on ultrasound and/or fetal MRI, and whether or not an amniocentesis had been performed.

We also noted information about the term and route of delivery, as well as the biometry at birth (presence or absence of congenital microcephaly or intrauterine growth retardation (IUGR)).

3.2.4. Clinical data

3.2.4.1. Anamnestic data

The referring department and the reason for consultation were noted. We also specified the presence or absence of neonatal hypotonia, feeding difficulties, psychomotor delay (motor delay, language delay), intellectual disability (ID), epilepsy and/or behavioural problems. We concluded that the child had psychomotor developmental delay according to the criteria in appendix 3. The presence or absence of an ID and its degree were communicated to us by the referring services.

3.2.4.2. Physical and paraclinical data

In this chapter, we set out the details of the physical examination carried out at the first consultation. We noted measurements (weight, height and head circumference), facial dysmorphia, musculoskeletal abnormalities, dermatological abnormalities, and abnormalities in neurological, cardiopulmonary, abdominal and urogenital examinations. New signs revealed during follow-up or by complementary or specialised examinations were also noted.

- Growth: Measurements were based on growth curves for age and sex.
- Facial dysmorphia: Dysmorphic features have been identified by a dysmorphological geneticist.
- Musculoskeletal abnormalities: Presence or absence of limb abnormalities or other musculoskeletal abnormalities revealed by the examination and/or bone X-rays.
- Dermatological abnormalities: Presence or absence of skin or appendage abnormalities and dermatoglyphic abnormalities.
- Neurological abnormalities: We noted abnormalities of tone, reflexes and balance.
- Behavioural problems: observed during consultations and/or confirmed by a specialist child psychiatry examination.

- Neurosensory abnormalities: detected by specialist ophthalmological and ENT (ear, nose and throat) examinations.

- Cardiovascular abnormalities: Presence or absence of abnormalities noted on cardiac auscultation and/or observed on cardiac ultrasound.

- Digestive anomalies: presence or absence of abdominal anomalies such as umbilical hernia, omphalocele or other anomalies revealed by the examination or abdominal imaging.

- Urogenital anomalies: Presence or absence of abnormalities of the external genitalia on clinical examination or other abnormalities of the urinary system or internal genitalia revealed by abdomino-pelvic ultrasound.

3.2.5. Brain MRI data

From the brain MRI report, we were able to answer these three questions:

- Is agenesis of the corpus callosum complete or partial? For partial agenesis, the agenesis segment was also specified.

- Are there any indirect signs associated with and/or indicative of agenesis of the corpus callosum? We have specified the type(s) of these indirect signs.

- Is agenesis of the corpus callosum isolated or associated with other brain anomaly(ies)? We have specified the type(s) of these anomaly(ies).

3.2.6. Genetic study

3.2.6.1. Cytogenetic study

We specified the results of the karyotype on amniotic fluid or blood lymphocytes from our patients. We also noted the results of molecular cytogenetic techniques (FISH (fluorescent *in situ* hybridisation) or ACPA (chromosome analysis on DNA chips)) carried out on some of our patients.

3.2.6.2. Molecular study

We have noted the targeted molecular biology analyses carried out on some of our patients.

4. DIAGNOSTIC ORIENTATION

All cases were presented at least once for diagnostic discussion at consultation meetings of the Congenital and Hereditary Diseases Department at Charles Nicolle Hospital in Tunis.

We also carried out a search on "Phenomizer-Orphanet" (http://compbio.charite.de/phenomizer/) for all the files [Appendix 4: Example of Phenomizer search results]. This is a web-based application used to guide clinical diagnosis in human genetics based on a search for similarity between the patient's phenotype and all known syndromes. The keywords are entered using the HPO (*The Human Phenotype Ontology*) nomenclature. We checked the similarity with the diagnoses mentioned by consulting the corresponding clinical tables in the following online databases:

- PubMed (www.ncbi.nlm.nih.gov/pubmed/)
- Orphanet: is a portal on rare diseases for the general public (www.orpha.net).
- OMIM (*Online Mendelian Inheritance in* Man®): is a catalogue of all known diseases of genetic origin in humans, linking them to the appropriate genes (www.omim.org).

5. STATISTICAL ANALYSIS

The data were entered using Microsoft Office Excel 2016. Statistical analysis of the data was carried out using IBM SPSS Statistics (*Statistical Package for the Social Sciences*) version 23 (free version).

For qualitative variables, we calculated absolute frequencies and relative frequencies (percentage). For quantitative variables, we calculated the means, medians and standard deviations and determined the extreme values. The qualitative variables were analysed using either the $\chi 2$ test or Fisher's exact test, depending on the theoretical numbers in the cross-tabulations.

Comparisons of quantitative variables between groups were made using either the Student's t-test (when the variable of interest was Gaussian) or a non-parametric test (Mann-Whitney-Wilcoxon test).

6. BIBLIOGRAPHIC RESEARCH AND BIBLIONET

The bibliographic search was carried out using the PubMed and Google scholar search engines. The keywords used were : *Agenesis of corpus callosum*, *Partial or complete*, *causes*, *intellectual disability*, *behaviour disorders*, *autism*, *genetic counseling* (www.hetop.eu).

The references were processed by ZOTERO (www.zotero.org) and cited in the text using this software.

7. ETHICAL CONSIDERATIONS

This work was carried out in compliance with ethical rules. The data were collected in compliance with professional secrecy. The patients' legal representatives gave their consent for the collection of personal data [Appendix 5].

8. CONFLICT OF INTEREST

We declare that there is no conflict of interest in this work.

Results

RESULTS

1. EPIDEMIOLOGICAL PROFILE

1.1. Description of the study population

Our study included 47 cases of agenesis of the corpus callosum collected over a period of 16 years, from January 2002 to December 2018 in the Department of Congenital and Hereditary Diseases at Charles Nicolle Hospital in Tunis.

1.2 Breakdown by gender

Of the 47 patients, 25 were male and 22 female, with a sex *ratio* (M/F) of 1.1.

1.3. Breakdown by age at first consultation

The median age at first consultation was 1.75 years [0.58; 7.41]. The extremes of age ranged from three days to 20 years. The age distribution of our study population is shown in Figure 1.

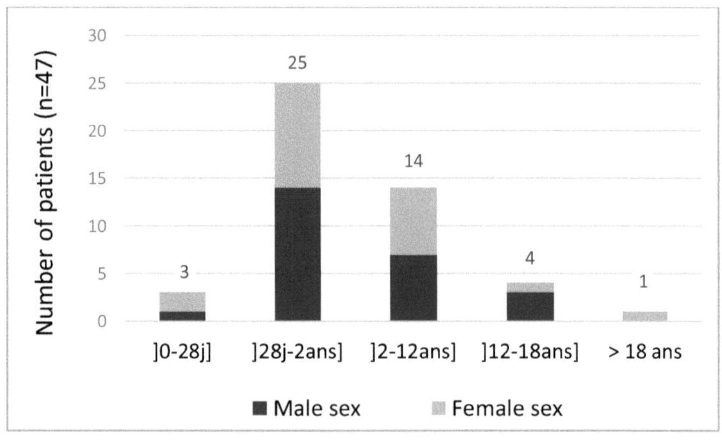

Figure 1*Distribution of patients with agenesis of the corpus callosum by age at first consultation.*

1.4. Breakdown by parents' geographical origin

Around 65% (27/42) of the parents came from the north of Tunisia, 63% (17/27) from the north-west [Figure 2].

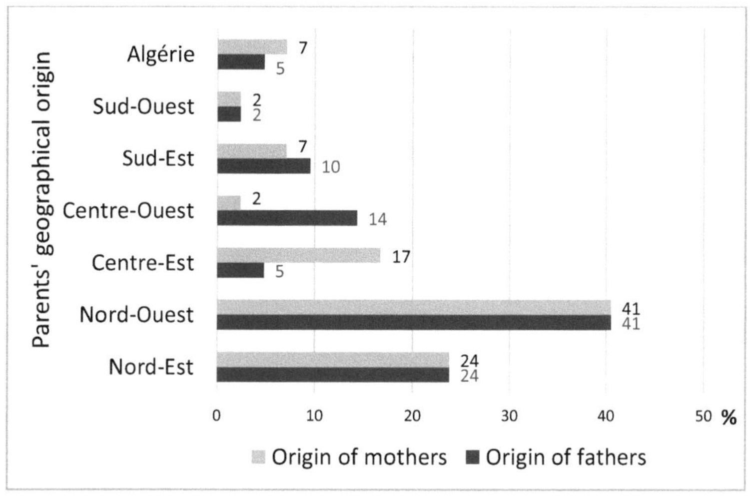

Figure 2*Distribution of patients with agenesis of the corpus callosum according to the geographical origin of the parents.*

1.5. Inbreeding

Consanguinity was noted in 38% (17/45) of cases.

1.6. Family history

1.6.1. History of corpus callosum anomalies in siblings

A history of corpus callosum anomaly in the siblings was found in approximately 24% (11/45) of cases. Among these anomalies, complete (5/11) or partial (5/11) agenesis was found in more than 90% of cases. A sibling history of hypoplasia of the corpus callosum was noted in only one patient [Figure 3].

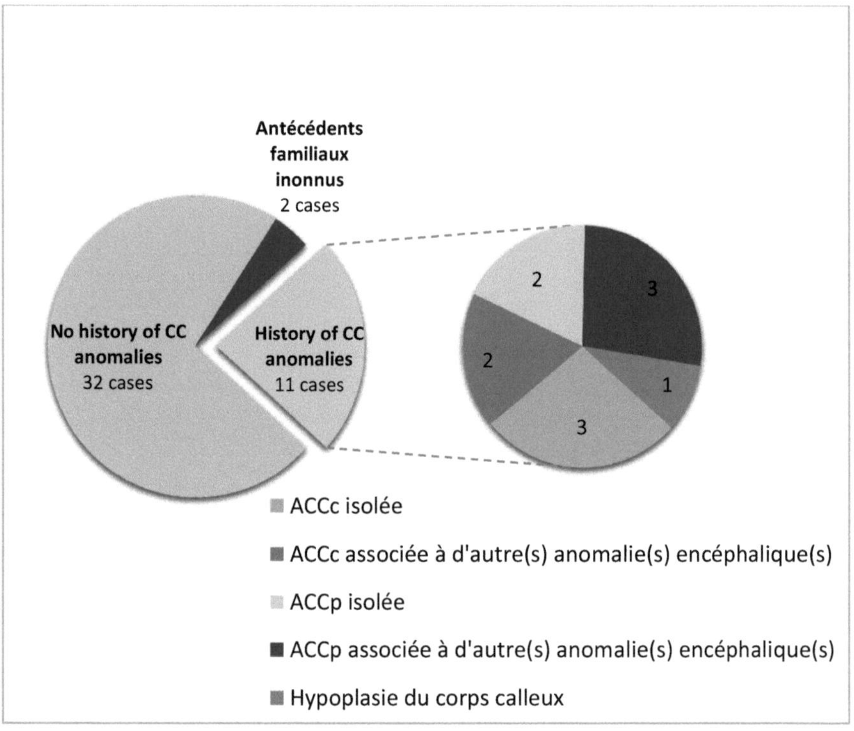

Figure 3*Sibling history of corpus callosum anomalies in patients with ACC.*

(CC: Corpus Callosum, ACC: Agenesis of the Corpus Callosum, complete (ACCc) or partial (ACCp)).

We have a total of 47 patients from 43 unrelated families with 6 familial forms of agenesis of the corpus callosum. Of these familial forms, it was only possible to examine all the index cases (2 cases per family) in four families (F2, F30, F42 and F43). For the other two families (F23 and F25), only one child consulted a doctor and was included in our study.

1.6.2. Family history of neurological abnormalities

A family history of neurological abnormalities other than corpus callosum anomalies was found in around 38% (17/45) of cases. These were most often developmental disorders and/or intellectual disabilities (8/17). Neurosensory damage such as deafness or ophthalmological abnormalities (5/17), cerebral malformation other than of the corpus callosum (2/17), microcephaly (1/17) or behavioural problems (1/17) were also found [Figure 4]. Of these 17 patients, four had a sibling history of corpus callosum anomaly.

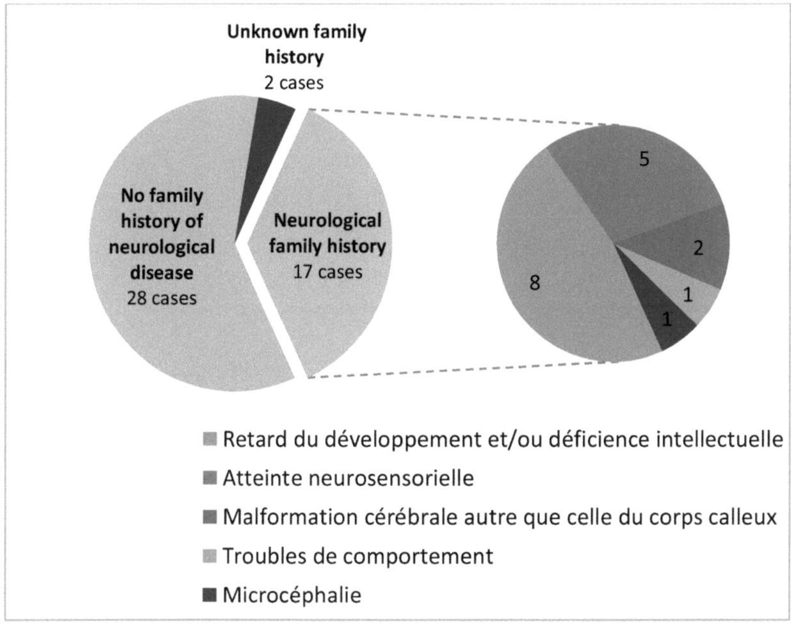

Figure 4*Family history of neurological abnormalities in patients with agenesis of the corpus callosum.*

2. MONITORING PREGNANCY AND CHILDBIRTH

2.1. Maternal age at conception

The mean maternal age was 30.7 years (±5.4). The extremes of age ranged from 22 to 42 years. Twenty-five per cent (11/44) of the mothers were aged 35 or over, including three aged over 40.

2.2. Special features of pregnancy

A well-monitored pregnancy was noted in 88% (37/42) of cases. Pregnancy follow-up data were missing in five cases.

A pregnancy induced by *in vitro* fertilisation (IVF) with a mother aged 40 and a father aged 54 was noted.

In one case, the mother had taken drugs during pregnancy. The mother was a smoker and alcoholic who took an antiparkinsonian anticholinergic (Artane®) and amphetamine (Ecstasy).

2.3 Prenatal signs and prenatal diagnosis

Second trimester ultrasound was performed in 88% (37/42) of pregnancies, of which around 32% (12/37) were performed by a doctor specialising in foetal imaging.

Prenatal signs were found in approximately 29% (12/42) of cases. These signs were revealed either by fetal ultrasound in the second trimester (6/12) or by ultrasound in the third trimester (6/12).

Ultrasound findings were confirmed by fetal MRI in five cases.

These signs were cerebral anomalies in 11 cases and hydramnios in the remaining case. The cerebral anomalies were agenesis of the corpus callosum (4 cases), isolated hydrocephalus (4 cases), unspecified cerebral malformation (2 cases) or microcephaly (1 case). CCA was isolated in one case, associated with hydrocephalus in two cases and associated with vermian agenesis with hydramnios in the remaining case [Figure 5].

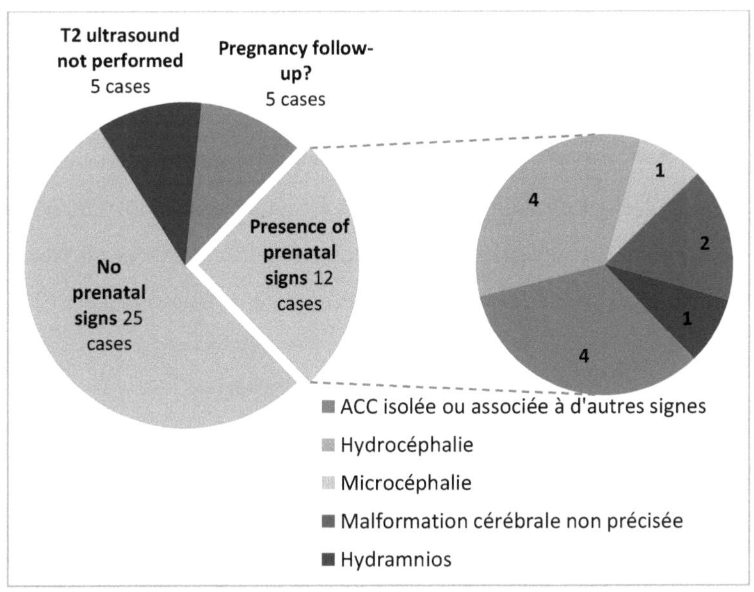

Figure 5*Prenatal signs in patients with agenesis of the corpus callosum (ACC).*

Among the 12 patients who had prenatal signs, a foetal karyotype on amniotic fluid was carried out in two cases and returned normal.

2.4. Delivery and birth biometrics

Ninety-six percent (45/47) of patients were born at term. The causes of premature delivery were a cervical defect in one case and hydramnios in the second. The route of delivery was specified in 35 cases, 69% of whom were born vaginally. Caesarean sections were performed for obstetric reasons (6/11), acute foetal distress (3/11) or for unspecified reasons (2/11).

Of the 47 cases, head circumference at birth was recorded in 25 cases and birth weight and height in 28 cases. Congenital microcephaly was found in 40% (10/25) of cases and IUGR in 25% (7/28). Of the cases with congenital microcephaly, 50% had IUGR.

3. CLINICAL STUDY

3.1 Reason for consultation and referring departments

In 74% (35/47) of cases, the reason for consultation was developmental delay, intellectual disability and/or cerebral malformation(s). The other reasons were hypotonia associated with dysmorphic features (4 cases), polymalformative syndrome (4 cases) or convulsive encephalopathy (4 cases) [Figure 6].

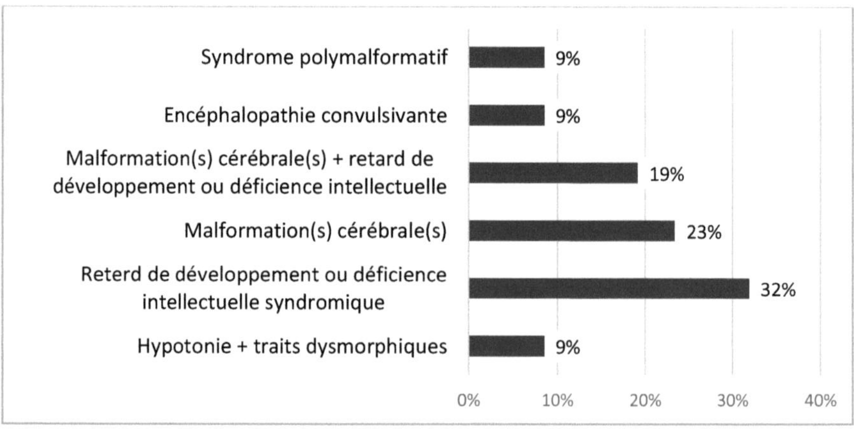

Figure 6*Reasons for consultation in patients with agenesis of the corpus callosum.*

Of the 47 patients, around 70% were referred by neuropaediatricians (20/47) or paediatricians (13/47). The other referring departments were: neonatology (6/47), child psychiatry (3/47), adult neurology (2/47) or basic health groups (3/47) [Figure 7].

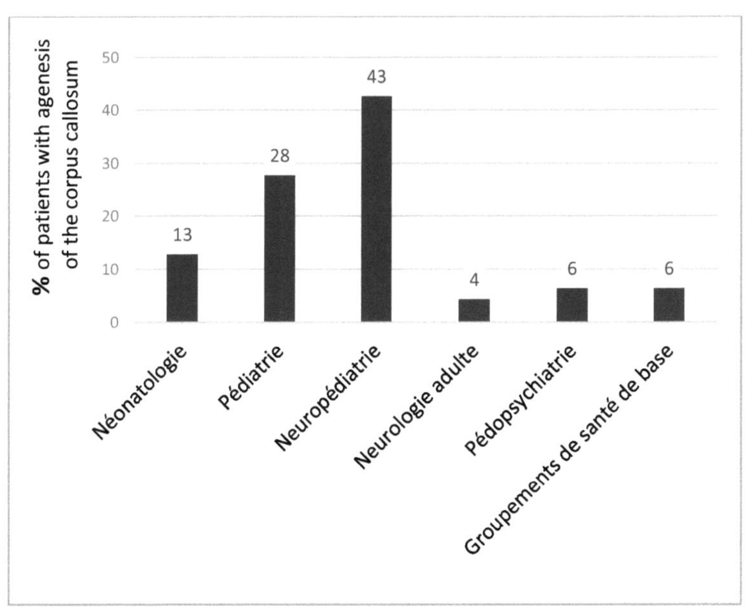

Figure 7*Distribution of patients with agenesis of the corpus callosum by referring department.*

3.2 Growth

About half the patients in our series had microcephaly and 15% had macrocephaly. The median head circumference at the first consultation was -1.85 DS [-3.4; 0 DS] with extremes ranging from -11.5 DS to +6.60 DS.

Delayed staturo-ponderal growth was noted in 37% of cases and advanced staturo-ponderal growth in 4%. The median height was -1.3 DS [-2.65 ;0 DS] with extremes ranging from -6.4 DS to +2.7 DS; and the median weight was 0 DS [-2.5 ;0 DS] with extremes ranging from -5.3 DS to +5 DS [Figure 8].

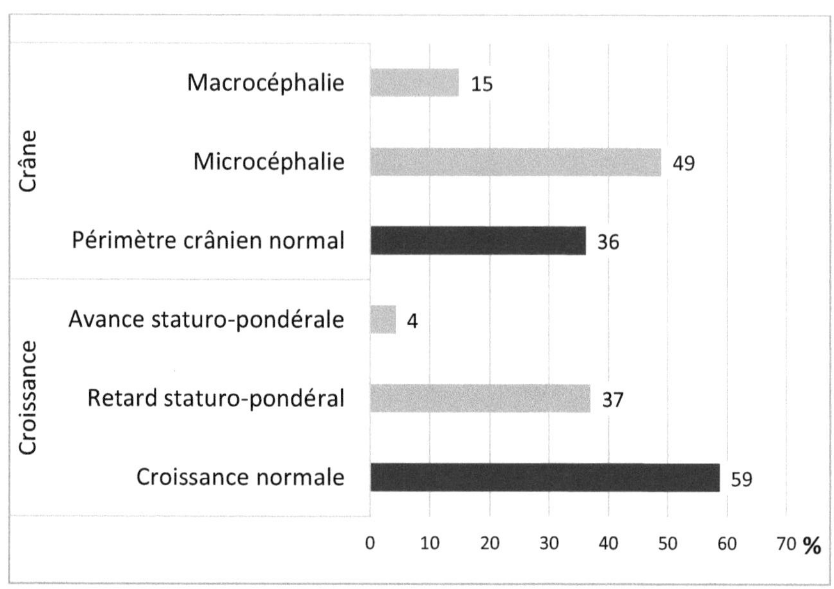

Figure 8*Distribution of patients with agenesis of the corpus callosum according to growth in height and weight and head circumference.*

3.3. Facial dysmorphia

Dysmorphic features were noted in approximately 94% (44/47) of patients in our series.

Among these patients, facial dysmorphia was suggestive of a particular syndrome in five cases: orofacial-digital syndrome type 1 in P7, Opitz syndrome type II (missense mutations of *SPECC1L*) in P9 and P33, Mowat-Wilson syndrome in P15 and microdeletion 15q24 syndrome in P19.

3.4. Musculoskeletal abnormalities

Limb anomalies were noted in 55% (26/47) of cases. Of these patients, 58% (15/26) had only one anomaly. The main limb anomalies are summarised in Table I.

*Table I*Limb anomalies in patients with agenesis of the corpus callosum (ACC).

Main limb anomalies	Frequency (n)	% of limb anomalies (n/40)	% among ACC patients (n/47)
Clinodactyly	11	28%	23%
Foot deformities	7	18%	15%
Camptodactyly	5	13%	11%
Post-axial hexadactyly	4	10%	9%
Thumb *adductus*	3	8%	6%
Ligament hyperlaxity	3	8%	6%
Overlapping toes	3	8%	6%
Brachydactyly	2	5%	4%
Partial syndactyly 2-3ème toes	2	5%	4%
Total	**40**	**100%**	*

* Several limb anomalies may be associated in the same patient.

Other musculoskeletal anomalies were noted in five patients. These anomalies included *pectus carinatum* or *excavatum* (5 cases), scoliosis (2 cases), asymmetric pelvis with *coxa valga* (1 case), delayed closure of the anterior fontanelle (1 case) and/or amyotrophy (2 cases).

3.5. Dermatological abnormalities

Skin and appendage abnormalities were noted in 17% (8/47) of cases. Nail dysplasia was found in 2 cases, hypertrichosis in 3 cases and/or pigmentation anomalies in 4 cases.

Dermatoglyph anomalies were noted in seven cases. These anomalies consisted of a single transverse palmar crease (4 cases), a supernumerary palmar crease (1 case) and finger palms (2 cases) with marked dermatoglyphs in one case.

3.6. Abnormalities of the external genitalia

Abnormalities of the external genitalia were present in 19% of cases. These anomalies were only found in male patients, i.e. 36% (9/25) of the boys in our series. These anomalies were cryptorchidism (8 cases) or phimosis (1 case). Cryptorchidism was associated in one case with hypogenitalism, in a second case with a buried penis and in a third case with sexual ambiguity.

3.7. Neurological abnormalities

3.7.1. Psychomotor development

Seventy-eight percent (36/46) of the patients in our series had a delay in motor acquisition and 85% (35/41) had a delay in language and/or absence of speech.

Among patients aged over three years (25 cases), intellectual disability was constant. It was mild in 2 cases, moderate in 7 and severe to profound in 5. The degree of ID was not specified in 11 cases.

3.7.2. Other neurological abnormalities

Tonus abnormalities were noted in 68% (32/47) of cases. Of these patients, 59% (19/32) had axial or global hypotonia and 41% (13/32) had axial hypotonia associated with peripheral hypertonia. Eating difficulties were noted in 6 patients in association with axial hypotonia. Pyramidal signs were found in 38% (18/47) of cases. Epilepsy was found in approximately 41% (19/47) of patients.

3.8. Behavioural problems

Of the 47 files examined, behavioural problems were noted in 10 patients: eight cases had features of autism spectrum disorder (ASD) (impaired social interaction, gestural stereotypies and/or hyperactivity), one case of polyphagia and one case of behavioural and conduct disorders such as aggression.

3.9. Neurosensory abnormalities

3.9.1. Ophthalmological abnormalities

Ophthalmological examination data were available in 35 of the 47 cases. Ophthalmological abnormalities were found in 69% (24/35) of cases. Several ophthalmological abnormalities were associated. Table II summarises the frequencies of these anomalies.

Table II*Ophthalmological abnormalities in patients with agenesis of the corpus callosum (ACC).*

Ophthalmological abnormalities	**Frequency** (n)	**% of ophthalmological anomalies** (n/41)	**% among ACC patients** (n/35)
Strabismus	11	27%	31%
Reduced visual acuity	8	20%	23%
Microphthalmia	5	12%	14%
Bilateral congenital cataract	4	10%	11%
Nystagmus	3	7%	9%
Ptosis	3	7%	9%
Congenital glaucoma	2	5%	6%
Optical atrophy	2	5%	6%
Retinal detachment	1	2%	3%
Luxation of the lens	1	2%	3%
Parafoveolar atrophy	1	2%	3%
Total	**41**	**100%**	*

* Several ophthalmological anomalies may be associated in the same patient.

3.9.2 Hearing impairment

Of the 47 cases examined, ENT examinations were carried out in 27 patients. Unilateral or bilateral deafness was found in 22% of cases (6/27).

3.10. Other associated congenital malformations

3.10.1. Cardiovascular malformations

Cardiac ultrasound was performed in 17 patients and revealed abnormalities in 4: one case of atrial septal defect (P21), one case of ventricular septal defect (P42), one case of patent ductus arteriosus with patent foramen ovale (P44) and one case of valvular pulmonary narrowing (P23).

3.10.2. Urogenital and digestive malformations

An umbilical hernia was found in two cases (P9 and P10). It was associated with an omphalocele in one case (P9) [Figure 9]. Abdomino-pelvic ultrasound was performed in 21 cases. Malformations were found in two cases: a case of uterus dysmorphic for age (P37) and a case of right renal duplicity with a left pelvic kidney (P19).

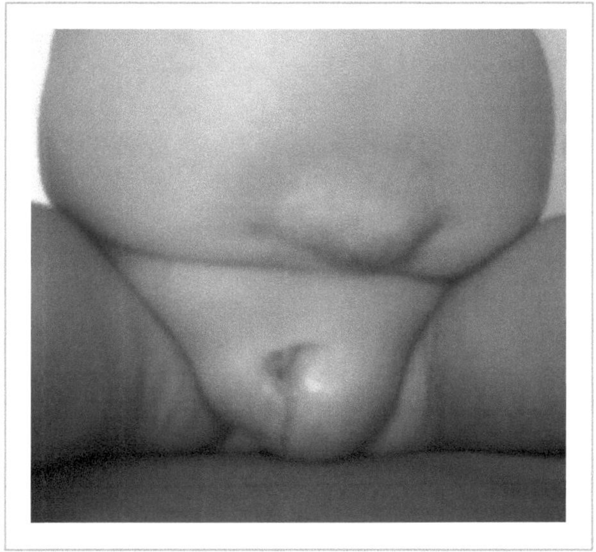

Figure 9*Umbilical hernia and omphalocele in P9.*

4. BRAIN MRI DATA

4.1. ACC: full or partial distribution

Among the files examined, 64% (30/47) of the ACCs were complete and 36% (17/47) were partial.

Among the partial agenesis cases, the segment of the corpus callosum affected was specified in 11 cases: the beak (1 case), the body (1 case), the splenium (3 cases) or the posterior part/body and splenium (6 cases) [Figure 10].

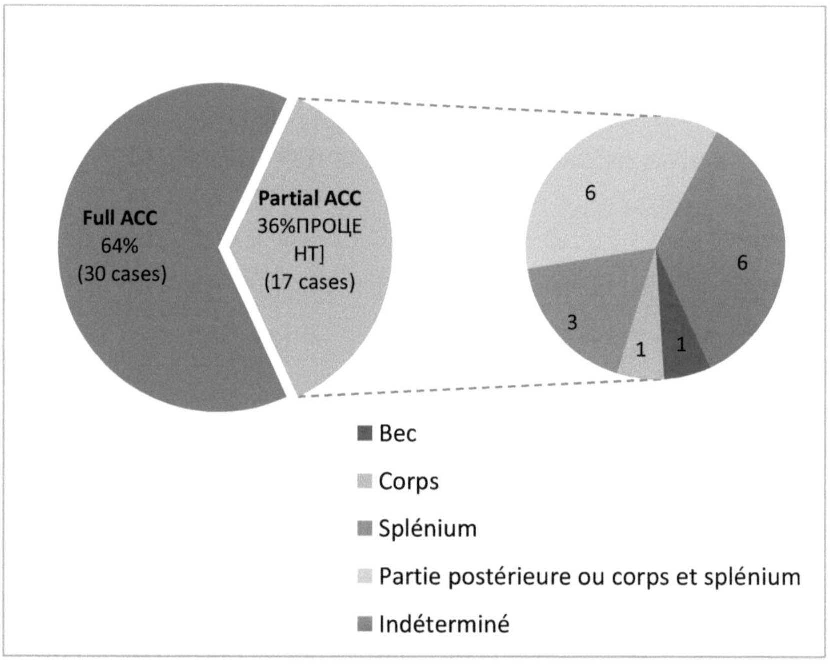

Figure 10*Distribution of complete or partial agenesis of the corpus callosum with the different agenesis segments.*

Clinical variability according to the type of CCA (complete or partial) is summarised in Table III.

Table III*Clinical variability according to the type of agenesis of the corpus callosum (complete or partial).*

Clinical picture		**ACC complete (%)**	**Partial ACC (%)**	**p-value**
Personal History	Prenatal signs	29	25	1
	Congenital microcephaly	35	50	0,667
	IUGR	35	9	0,191
Growth	Abnormal growth in height and weight	48	29	0,210
	Abnormal cranial perimeter	63	65	0,925
Neurological signs	Engine delay	72	88	0,282
	Language delay	84	88	1
	Eating difficulties	31	8	0,196
	Epilepsy	52	24	0,073
Behavioural problems	Behavioural problems	17	38	0,159
	Autistic traits	13	25	0,415
Associated extra-cerebral anomalies	Facial dysmorphia	90	100	0,292
	Extremity abnormalities	53	65	0,449
	EMB anomalies	17	24	0,704
	Eye abnormalities	67	71	1
	Hearing problems	14	31	0,385
Brain MRI data	Indirect signs of ACC	93	80	0,544
	Associated brain abnormalities	53	65	0,449
Diagnosis evoked		40	41	0,938

ACC: agenesis of the corpus callosum, **IUGR:** intrauterine growth retardation, **EGO:** external genitalia.

4.2. Indirect signs of ACC

Of the 47 cases examined, the presence or absence of indirect signs of ACC was noted in 26 cases. These signs were present in 23 cases. Approximately 52% (12/23) of cases had only one indirect sign on MRI. These signs were divided into abnormalities of the lateral ventricles, abnormalities of the 3ème ventricle, Probst bands, abnormalities of the convolutions and/or abnormalities of the other commissures [Table IV].

Table IV *Indirect signs on MRI and their distribution according to the type of agenesis of the corpus callosum.*

Indirect signs of ACC on cerebral MRI		Full ACC	Partial ACC	Total
Lateral ventricles	Colpocephaly	5	1	6
	Temporal horn abnormalities	2	1	3
	Frontal horn abnormalities	2	0	2
	Anomalies of the ventricular carrefices	2	0	2
	Enlargement of the interventricular space or parallel appearance of the LVs	6	2	8
	Septal agenesis	1	1	2
Ascent of the third ventricle		2	2	4
Transtentorial hydrocephalus		3	3	6
Probst strips		1	1	2
Circonvolutions	Absence of the cingulate *gyrus*	1	0	1
	Ocular dysplasia	1	0	1
	Temporal dysplasia	0	1	1
Other commissures	Agenesis of the anterior commissure	2	1	3

	Hypoplasia or malrotation of the hippocampi	2	3	5
Total		**30**	**16**	**46**

ACC: agenesis of the corpus callosum, **LV:** lateral ventricles.

4.3. Brain abnormalities associated with ACC

Agenesis of the corpus callosum was associated with other brain anomaly(ies) in 57% (27/47) of cases [Table V]. These were :

- Migration or gyration abnormalities: Cortical and/or subcortical atrophy (5 cases), lissencephaly (3 cases), polymicrogyria (2 cases), schizencephaly (2 cases) and/or nodular heterotopia (1 case).
- White matter abnormalities (4 cases)
- Arachnoid cysts (2 cases) or inter-hemispheric cysts (2 cases)
- Posterior fossa anomalies: Dandy-Walker malformation (4 cases), dilatation of the fourth ventricle and/or large cistern (4 cases), Joubert malformation (2 cases) and/or other cerebellar anomalies (2 cases).
- Ocular anomalies: one case of retinal detachment and one case of lens dislocation in the posterior chamber.

Table V*Associated brain anomalies and their distribution according to the type of agenesis of the corpus callosum (ACC).*

Associated brain abnormalities	Full ACC	Partial ACC	Total
Migration and/or gyration abnormalities	9	4	13
White matter abnormalities	4	0	4
Arachnoid cysts	1	1	2
Interhemispheric cyst	1	1	2
Abnormalities of the posterior fossa	7	5	12
Eye abnormalities	1	1	2

Total	23	12	35

Among patients with complete agenesis, 53% (16/30) had associated encephalic anomalies, and among patients with partial agenesis 65% (11/17) had other encephalic anomalies.

Sixty-six percent (23/35) of the associated signs were found in patients with complete agenesis and the remaining 34% (12/35) were found in patients with partial agenesis.

Clinical variability according to the presence or absence of encephalic abnormality(ies) is summarised in Table VI.

Table VI*Clinical variability according to the presence or absence of associated encephalic anomaly(ies).*

Clinical picture		**Without associated brain abnormalities (%)**	**With associated brain abnormalities (%)**	**p-value**
Personal History	Prenatal signs	26	28	0,113
	Congenital microcephaly	37,5	41	1
	IUGR	18	29	0,668
Growth	Abnormal growth in height and weight	50	35	0,193
	Abnormal cranial perimeter	45	78	0,082
Neurological signs	Engine delay	70	81	0,292
	Language delay	75	74	0,396
	Eating difficulties	20	22	1
	Epilepsy	30	50	0,172
Behavioural problems	Behavioural problems	35	17	0,274
	Autistic traits	25	13	0,415
	Facial dysmorphia	95	93	1

Associated extra-cerebral anomalies	Extremity abnormalities	50	63	0,374
	EMB anomalies	15	22	0,712
	Ocular abnormalities	61,5	73	0,707
	Hearing problems	9	31	0,349
Brain MRI data	Full ACC	70	59	0,449
	Partial ACC	30	41	0,449
	Indirect signs of ACC on MRI	83	93	0,580
Diagnosis evoked		25	52	0,079

ACC: agenesis of the corpus callosum, **IUGR:** intrauterine growth retardation, **EGO:** external genitalia.

5. GENETIC STUDY

5.1. Cytogenetic study

5.1.1. Karyotype

The karyotype performed on blood lymphocytes (45/47) or amniotic fluid (2/47) was normal in all cases.

5.1.2. Fluorescent *in situ* hybridization

Fluorescent *in situ* hybridisation (FISH) was performed in seven cases, i.e. 19% of patients. The indication, probe used and results are summarised in Table VII.

Table VII *FISH* ***analysis of*** *seven patients with agenesis of the corpus callosum.*

Patient	Diagnostic suspicion	Probe used in FISH	Results
P20	Miller-Dieker syndrome (MDS)	*LIS1* locus-specific VYSIS ISL	Absence of microdeletion compatible with MDS
P21			
P45			

P13	22q11.2 microdeletion syndrome	*TBX1* locus-specific probe	Absence of microdeletion of the TBX1 locus
P33	G/BBB Opitz syndrome in the autosomal dominant form		
P9	Microduplication syndrome 7q36.3	RP11-69O3 at the *SHH* locus in 7q36.3	Absence of microduplication of the SHH locus
	Mosaic of Trisomy 13	LSI 13 specific to the *RB1* locus in 13q14	No aneuploidy of chromosome 13
	Wolf-Hirschhorn syndrome (SWH)	VYSIS WHS13 LSI specific to the *WHSC1* locus at 4p16.3	Absence of microdeletion compatible with SWH
P43	Mosaic of Trisomy 8	VYSIS CEP8 LSI specific to the D8Z1 locus at 8p11.1-q11.1	Presence of a small trisomy 8 mosaic (5%)

FISH: fluorescent *in situ* hybridisation, ***LIS1***: Lissencephaly-1, ***TBX1***: T-box 1, ***SHH***: sonic hedgehog, ***RB1***: RB transcriptional corepressor 1, ***WHSC1***: Wolf-Hirschhorn syndrome candidate 1.

5.1.3. Chromosome analysis on a DNA chip

ACPA was performed in a patient with syndromic intellectual disability and returned normal.

5.2 Molecular study

The diagnosis of fragile X-linked syndrome by amplification of CGG triplets was not accepted in three male patients (P28, P42, P47). Spinal muscular atrophy syndrome was ruled out in P2 and Prader-Willi syndrome in P32. Sequencing of the *NPHP1* gene was normal in P44 and P45.

6. DIAGNOSTIC ORIENTATION

A diagnosis was evoked in approximately 40% (19/47) of cases. Table VIII summarises the arguments that led to this diagnostic orientation for each of these patients.

*Table VIII**Diagnosis of 19 patients with agenesis of the corpus callosum.*

	Patient	Diagnosis evoked	Elements in favour diagnosis	Against diagnosis
(F2)	P2	Cockayne syndrome in its classic form (CS I)	- Related and asymptomatic parents, presence of family cases - Bilateral congenital cataract and microphthalmia - Low weight and microcephaly - Severe developmental delay - Axial hypotonia contrasting with peripheral hypertonia - ACC (splenium)	- No deafness, pigmentary retinopathy or photosensitivity - No peripheral neuropathy - No other brain abnormalities
(F2)	P3			
(F6)	P7	Type 1 orofacial-digital syndrome	- Female sex - Evocative DF [Figure 9 page 18] with gingival brake and ogival palate - Polydactyly - Delayed development - Heterotopy, MDW, complete ACC	- No microcephaly - No small size - No renal cysts
(F8)	P9	*SPECC1L* syndrome *(Opitz G/BBB type II syndrome)*	- Evocative DF [Figure 10 page 18] with ogival palate and bifid uvula - Complete ACC and subcortical atrophy - Developmental delay and ID - Umbilical hernia and omphalocele [Figure 13 page 24].	- presence of microcephaly
	P14 (F13)	Neonatal Cockayne syndrome (CS II)	- Asymptomatic relatives, family history of neurological impairment - Neonatal hypotonia and developmental delay - Microcephaly and progressive RC postnatally	- No deafness, pigmentary retinopathy or photosensitivity -No signs of peripheral

		- Bilateral congenital cataract and microphthalmia - Axial hypotonia contrasting with peripheral hypertonia and epilepsy - ACCc, SB anomaly - Bilateral cryptorchidism	neurological damage - No other brain abnormalities
P15 (F14)	Mowat-Wilson syndrome	- Evocative DF [Figure 11 page 19]. - Delayed development - Epilepsy, spasticity and ACC - Stereotypies	- No microcephaly or small stature - Cardiovascular and intestinal malformations?
P19 (F18)	15q24 microdeletion syndrome	- Ante-natal onset CR and microcephaly - Evocative DF [Figure 12 page 19]. - Brachydactyly and hyperlaxity - Hypotonia and developmental delay - Behavioural problems, deafness - ACC and frontal hypoplasia	- Presence of renal malformations
P20 (F19)	Serine deficiency	- Congenital microcephaly and IUGR - Bilateral congenital cataract - Epilepsy and spastic tetraparesis - Deafness, Developmental delay - Ichthyosis, large ears and short neck - ACC, lissencephaly, MDW	- Unrelated parents

P22 (F21)	Tubulinopathy (*TUBB2B* mutation)	- Severe PMR - Epilepsy - ACC and perisylvian polymicrogyria - Optical atrophy	- Macrocephaly (hydrocephalus) - Peripheral hypertonia
P23 (F22)	Tubulinopathy	- RPM, DI, peripheral hypertonia - Epilepsy - Microcephaly - Optical atrophy, visual impairment - ACC, cortico-subcortical atrophy	- Presence of cardiovascular and skeletal abnormalities
P24 (F23)	Tubulinopathy (*TUBB4A* mutation)	- Microcephaly and short stature - VI oculomotor paralysis - ACC, global cortical atrophy, demyelinating leukoencephalopathy	
P31 (F30)	Borjeson-Forssman-Lehmann syndrome	- ID in 2 brothers and a maternal cousin of the mother: heredity compatible with X-linked recessive transmission - Neonatal hypotonia, developmental delay, ID and epilepsy - Obesity and short stature - Palpebral ptosis - Behavioural problems - Bilateral cryptorchidism in P32	- ACC rare sign
P32 (F30)			
P33 (F31)	*SPECC1L* syndrome (Opitz G/BBB type II syndrome)	- Evocative FD: prominent forehead, hypertelorism, oblique lower and lateral FPs - Developmental delay and ID - Full ACC	- Epilepsy - Absence of other midline anomalies

P34 (F32)	Seckel syndrome	- Consanguinity, family history of dwarfism (4 cases) - Severe growth retardation and microcephaly - Delayed development - Full ACC	- Behavioural problems - Bone assessment?
P37 (F35)	Joubert syndrome	- Appearance of a molar tooth with vermilion hypoplasia, partial ACC - Macrocephaly - Hypotonia and RPM - Epilepsy - Post-axial hexadactyly	- No respiratory problems - Kidney and eye damage? - No inbreeding
P43 (F41)	Mosaic of Trisomy 8	- Full ACC - Developmental delay and ID - Left corneal opacity - Skeletal anomalies - Finger palms, marked dermatoglyphs, excess skin in the armpits	
P44 (F42) P45 (F42)	Joubert syndrome	- Consanguinity - Macrocephaly **At P44 :** - Molar tooth appearance with inferior vermian agenesis and superior dysplasia, V4 dilatation, hippocampal malrotation, thalamic fusion and ACC - Hypotonia and RPM - PCA and patent foramen ovale **At P45 :** - Hexadactyly - MDW, ACCc with V3 dilatation and VL spacing, polymicrogyria	- No respiratory problems - Kidney and eye damage?

ACC: agenesis of the corpus callosum, **DF**: facial dysmorphia, **ID**: intellectual disability, **FP**: cleft palate, **MDW**: Dandy-Walker malformation, **RC**: growth retardation, **RPM**: psychomotor retardation.

7. CONSEIL GENETIQUE

Genetic counselling could not be given to the families of patients without a diagnosis.

For patients for whom a diagnosis was evoked, genetic counselling based on the mode of transmission of this pathology was given:

- For autosomal recessive (AR) diseases (Cockayne, Seckel, Joubert syndromes, serine deficiency and certain tubulinopathies), we explained that the risk of recurrence with each pregnancy is 25%. A prenatal diagnosis (PND) will therefore be indicated in the event of molecular confirmation.

- In the case of autosomal dominant (AD) diseases (*SPECC1L* missense mutation syndrome, Mowat-Wilson syndrome, 15q24 microdeletion syndrome and certain tubulinopathies), which occur in patients of apparently healthy parents and which tend to be *de novo*, we have explained that the risk of recurrence is low. However, a PND should be considered if the diagnosis is confirmed, given the risk of geminal mosaicism.

- For X-linked dominant diseases (XLD) (oro-facio-digital syndrome type 1), which occur in patients of apparently healthy parents, the risk of recurrence, although low, is difficult to predict, not only because of the risk of germline mosaicism, but also because of the bias of X chromosome inactivation in the mother and the possibility of incomplete penetrance and variable expressivity of dominant diseases. If the diagnosis is confirmed, PND may be proposed.

- For X-linked recessive (XLR) diseases (Borjeson-Forssman-Lehmann and Joubert syndromes), the risk of recurrence for male offspring is 50% (daughters will be carriers in half the cases). If the diagnosis is confirmed, PND will therefore be indicated for subsequent pregnancies if the foetus is male.

For all these patients, and because of the lack of diagnostic confirmation, ultrasound monitoring was proposed for subsequent pregnancies.

Discussion

DISCUSSION

Our descriptive and retrospective study determined the clinical and epidemiological characteristics of 47 cases of agenesis of the corpus callosum collected over a period of 16 years in the Department of Congenital and Hereditary Diseases at Charles Nicolle Hospital in Tunis.

As we only see symptomatic patients at our clinic, we were unable to recruit asymptomatic patients with incidental findings of ACC on brain imaging.

To our knowledge, this is the first epidemiological and clinical study of agenesis of the corpus callosum in Tunisia.

Thanks to the clinical study of each patient, we were able to orientate the diagnosis in more than 37% (16/43) of families and provide appropriate genetic counselling despite the absence of cytogenetic or molecular confirmation.

However, we noted some missing data, which can be explained on the one hand by the retrospective nature of our study (the data refer in particular to the prenatal period), and on the other hand by the lack of follow-up. This early cessation of follow-up prevented us from collecting certain data, particularly concerning intellectual disability.

1. EPIDEMIOLOGICAL PROFILE

1.1. Prevalence

Agenesis of the corpus callosum is the most common congenital cerebral malformation. Synthesis of studies based on neonatal and prenatal imaging data has suggested that ACC occurs in at least 1/4000 live births (6-8). This prevalence is higher in populations with developmental disorders ranging from 230 to 600/10000 (3,7). However, the exact prevalence of this malformation remains difficult to determine due to selection bias in the series reported. In addition, CCA is not always diagnosed in the ante-natal period, and its expression is variable and may be virtually silent in the first few years of life (3,5). The best data available are from two studies which determined the prevalence of ACC by referring to national registers of congenital malformations. The first was a Californian study conducted over 20 years, which found a prevalence of 1.4 cases per 10,000 live births, and the second was an Italian study conducted over 34 years, which found a prevalence of 2.1 cases per 10,000 live births (8,9).

In Tunisia, we have no data on the prevalence of agenesis of the corpus callosum in our population. To determine this prevalence, a national register of congenital malformations should be set up.

1.2 Breakdown by gender

In our series, there was a very slight predominance of males, with a *sex* ratio (M/F) of 1.1. In the literature, the *sex* ratio varies from 1.25 to 1.68 depending on the study (4,8-10).

This distribution in favour of the male sex could firstly be attributed to a socio-cultural bias, since the women affected were more often kept at home rather than institutionalized, with a greater level of consultation for the male subjects. In addition, the absence of a strong *sex-ratio* bias would reflect the complexity of corpus callosum development, with the involvement of several genes on several chromosomes (4).

1.3. Age distribution

All age groups were represented in our series, with a predominance of patients aged between 28 days and 2 years.] However, despite the 16-year inclusion period, it is important to note that 51% (24/47) of our patients consulted us only once, and half of them were less than three years old. Of the remaining patients (23/47) who had consulted at least twice, 39% (9/23) were under three years of age.

1.4. Breakdown by parents' geographical origin

All regions of Tunisia were represented in our study. Around 65% of our patients were from the north. This predominance could be explained by the population density and the proximity of these regions to our department. In addition, the creation of new genetic services in the centre of the country could explain the low frequency of consultants from central and southern Tunisia.

1.5. Inbreeding

Consanguinity was noted in 38% of cases. This figure is higher than the rate of consanguinity in the general population in Tunisia, which is 29.8%. (11). A second study carried out in the United Arab Emirates (UAE) also found a high rate of consanguinity (44%) in a cohort of ACC (12). This figure should be interpreted with caution, bearing in mind that the rate of consanguinity in the general population in the UAE varies from 39% to 54.2%. (13).

Consanguinity is thought to be a risk factor for ACC, which is one of the autosomal recessive transmission syndromes (14). Indeed, the involvement of consanguinity in the occurrence of autosomal recessive transmission diseases was previously established in Tunisia (15).

1.6. Family history

1.6.1. History of corpus callosum anomalies in siblings

The majority of patients with a sibling history of CC anomaly are from consanguineous marriages (8/11). These data provide a further argument in favour of the involvement of consanguinity in the occurrence of recessive diseases.

1.6.2. Family history of neurological abnormalities

The co-occurrence in the same family of ACC with developmental disorders, neurosensory anomalies or other encephalic anomalies could be due to the variable expressivity of the same disease. In most of the syndromes involved, the penetrance of ACC is incomplete. (2). This variable expressivity could also be explained by the involvement of other genetic and/or environmental factors (1).

2. MONITORING PREGNANCY AND CHILDBIRTH

2.1. Maternal age at conception

In our series, the mean maternal age at conception (30.7 ± 5.4 years) was slightly higher than the mean age of parturients in Tunisia, which is 28.8 ± 5.5 years. In addition, the frequency of mothers of advanced age, greater than or equal to 35 years, was higher than that of the general population (25% *versus* 17%). (16).

Glass et *al* also noted this predominance of advanced maternal age in patients with ACC and also noted that the risk of ACC linked to a chromosomal anomaly was six times higher in mothers aged over 40 years. (9).

These findings are largely linked to the higher risk - at least fourfold - of chromosomal abnormalities in mothers aged 35 and over, compared with mothers aged 25 to 29 (17,18). This risk is linked to recombination and chromosomal disjunction anomalies during female meiosis (19).

In addition, the accumulation of DNA damage with age could increase the risk of *de novo* mutations.

However, of the 11 cases in mothers aged 35 and over at conception, an autosomal dominant disease was suggested in only one case (Opitz syndrome in P33) and a chromosomal abnormality was not suggested in any case in our series.

2.2. Special features of pregnancy

Data concerning the consumption of alcohol or other toxic substances, the onset of gestational diabetes, antenatal infections and the use of medically assisted reproduction (MAP) were not detailed enough in the files to be analysed, although they are considered in the literature to be linked to abnormalities of the corpus callosum. (1).

One case in our series (P12) was found to have taken toxic drugs during pregnancy. The mother was a smoker and alcoholic who took an antiparkinsonian anticholinergic and amphetamine. In this patient, the clinical picture was not suggestive of a particular genetic syndrome, which argues in favour of the environmental origin of agenesis of the corpus callosum.

The teratogenic and neurotoxic effects of alcohol are well established, and its association with abnormalities in brain development has been described in several studies. Cerebral malformations are extremely variable, affecting all stages of development of the central nervous system. Cerebral volume reduction and CC malformations, such as agenesis or hypoplasia, are the two most frequent disorders reported in association with prenatal exposure to alcohol. (20-23). At the cellular level, ethanol appears to inhibit the *Sonic Hedgehog* pathway, modify retinoic acid activity levels, trigger a CamKII calcium-dependent pathway that antagonises Wnt pathway signalling, affect cytoskeletal dynamics and increase oxidative stress (24,25).

Despite prenatal exposure to alcohol, examination of our patient P12 did not reveal any facial dysmorphia suggestive of foetal alcohol syndrome or FAS (narrow cleft palpebras, flat, effaced philtrum, thin upper lip) or any microcephaly or growth retardation. However, the neurological impairment in this patient, combining CCA, epilepsy and developmental delay, could be classified as Fetal Alcohol Spectrum Disorder (FASD). (26). This isolated neurological impairment would thus be linked to the fact that the brain is the organ most affected by prenatal exposure to alcohol (23). The teratogenicity of alcohol is constant throughout the development of the central nervous system, and cerebral malformations can occur during embryogenesis or foetogenesis. There is therefore no specific period for alcohol neurotoxicity. On the other hand, facial malformations are more frequent in cases of alcohol consumption during the first trimester of pregnancy, given the inducing effect of the prosencephalon on the face and the development of the frontonasal bud. (27).

We were unable to determine the period of prenatal exposure to alcohol in P12 because he was adopted. In addition, other genetic or environmental factors may be involved in this patient's phenotype.

The effect of tobacco on foetal brain development has not been studied. However, exposure to tobacco in adults inhibits the expression of the genes needed to synthesise and maintain myelin. Tobacco could therefore contribute to the degeneration of white matter (28). The corpus callosum could be one of the main targets influenced by chronic smoking. In fact, there is a significant negative correlation between fatty acids in the whole of the CC and the amount of tobacco consumed (29,30). The involvement of tobacco in the development of ACC cannot be ruled out, and would need to be confirmed by exposure studies on animal models or by studies of large cohorts of children born to smoking mothers.

The effects of antiparkinsonian drugs and amphetamine on brain development have not been studied according to current data. In the absence of diagnostic guidance, P12's phenotype could be attributed to prenatal exposure to alcohol and/or tobacco.

Patient P42 resulted from an IVF-induced pregnancy with a mother aged 40 and a father aged 54. It is true that, to date, cohort studies on the follow-up of children born after MAP have been reassuring, but it remains to be seen whether the cellular stress caused by the manipulation of gametes and embryos *in vitro* could be the cause of a higher risk of epigenetic anomalies or foetal malformations. (31). Furthermore, the advanced age of the parents could be the cause of the occurrence of *de novo* mutations in P42.

2.3. Prenatal diagnosis

2.3.1 Fetal imaging

The corpus callosum begins to individualise at 12-14 weeks of pregnancy. The first portion of the CC to develop is the knee, then its growth follows a bidirectional rostro-caudal progression until 20 weeks when its structure is anatomically complete (1,7,32,33). It continues to grow in thickness during the 3 trimester and for the first two years of life. Myelination begins in the posterior part of the myelin at 2 months of age, and maturation continues into adulthood (1,34).

As a result, developmental abnormalities of the corpus callosum cannot be detected before 20 weeks gestational age. Consequently, prenatal diagnosis of CVA is essentially made by fetal ultrasound (FUS) in the second trimester (1,6,8).

The corpus callosum can be identified in a sagittal midline view of the foetal brain as a hypoechoic structure located between the cavity of the septum pellucidum and the cingulate *gyrus*, bounded by two echogenic lines. The pericallear artery, which develops in close association with the CC, can also serve as a useful ultrasound marker (35). An abnormal trajectory or biometry of this artery was recently proposed as an early (first trimester) ultrasound marker of abnormal CC development. In fact, the pericallear artery and its branches can be identified and measured from 11 weeks onwards. (36).

The diagnosis of CFA in FE is based on complete or partial non-visibility of the CC. However, the CC, which is physiologically very thin and not myelinated, is difficult to examine antenatally. Ultrasound diagnosis may be suggested by the presence of indirect signs, the most frequent being the absence of the septum pellucidum (SPC) cavity, the teardrop appearance of the lateral ventricles (LVs), the ascension of the 3ème ventricle, the asymmetric enlargement of the LVs, the widening of the interhemispheric fissure, and the radial arrangement of the medial convolutions (37,38) [Figure 11].

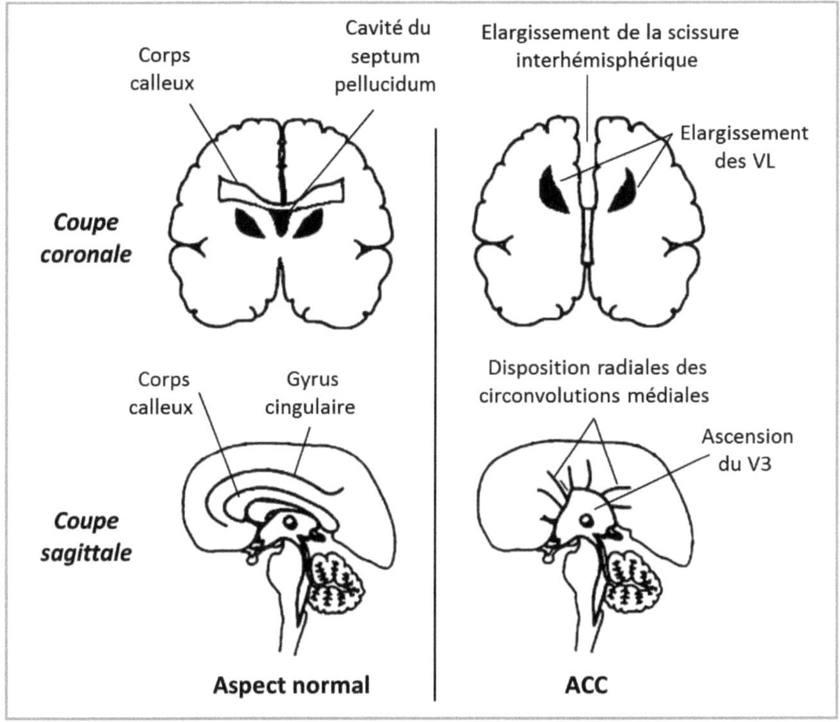

Figure 11*Schematic representation of the indirect signs of CCA on foetal ultrasound (Modified from (37)). (ACC: agenesis of the corpus callosum, LV: lateral ventricle, V3: 3ème ventricle)*

These indirect signs of callosal agenesis are inconstant and less marked when the agenesis is partial (38). For example, the absence of the septum pellucidum cavity is consistently found in complete agenesis, whereas it is only detected in about half of partial agenesis. However, the PSC is abnormal in appearance (wide and short) in the majority of the remaining cases of ACCp (38-40).

Because of its non-myelinated structure, visualisation of the CC is imperfect on FE, and fetal MRI is an additional imaging option when an abnormality is suspected on ultrasound (35,41).

MRI can be used to confirm the presence or absence of CCA and to more accurately characterise whether it is complete or partial. In fact, some studies have found 5-20% of false positives on ultrasound that are invalidated by MRI (32,42,43). MRI shows the indirect signs described on FE, as well as other signs such as Probst bands and abnormalities of the cingulate sulcus. In addition, MRI provides a better analysis of the white matter and improves the detection of cerebral anomalies associated with CFA, in particular gyration anomalies, heterotopias and cystic malformations. For example, 23% of brain abnormalities detected by MRI were not visualised by ultrasound (8).

The anomalies most frequently detected by fetal MRI are ventriculomegaly (78.6%), cortical malformations (53.6%), posterior fossa malformations (25%) and midline anomalies (10.7%). (41).

Fetal brain MRI is ideally performed between 26 and 30 weeks of pregnancy. Before 26ème weeks, the fetal brain is physiologically smooth, and after 31ème weeks, the reduction in pericerebral fluids can hamper its interpretation. Thus, although MRI confirms the diagnosis of CFA from 22 weeks of pregnancy, it does not detect associated gyration abnormalities at this stage, which are one of the factors affecting the neurological prognosis of the unborn child (44,45).

In our series, second trimester ultrasound was performed in the majority of cases (88%) but revealed abnormalities in only 16% (6/37) of cases. This low rate compared with that reported in the literature may be explained by the fact that second trimester ultrasound was not systematically performed by a doctor specialising in foetal imaging. The rate of diagnosis of CVA in the literature has increased from 60% to 90% thanks to second-trimester screening ultrasound, which has become systematic. (8).

Callous agenesis was visualised in one third of cases where anomalies were discovered antenatally (3 cases of ACCc and one case of ACCp) and was associated with other signs in 3 cases: an indirect sign (hydrocephalus) in two cases or encephalic anomalies (arachnoid cyst and vermian agenesis) in the remaining case. The other anomalies revealed by FE were microcephaly in one case and hydrocephaly in the remaining case. CCA was not detected prenatally in two patients, although fetal MRI was performed in one case. Callosal agenesis was partial in both cases, demonstrating the limitations of prenatal imaging in the diagnosis of pCCA.

Of the six patients with an anomaly detected on second-trimester FM, fetal MRI was performed in four patients and confirmed the anomalies detected on ultrasound.

Prenatal signs were also detected in six patients at third-trimester ultrasound, whereas second-trimester EF was normal in all of these cases.

In our series, morphological ultrasound in the second trimester, performed by a doctor specialising in foetal imaging, was performed in only 12 cases. This could be explained by socio-economic and health reasons: specialised ultrasound not available in basic health centres, centralisation of third-level maternity centres in large towns and the high cost of treatment in private facilities with a low rate of reimbursement by the national health insurance fund.

2.3.2. Aetiological diagnosis

Once callosal agenesis has been detected on foetal imaging, it is essential to determine whether it is isolated or associated, on which the prognosis will depend. An aetiological assessment must also be carried out. This should look for the presence or absence of a family history, the notion of consanguinity, any toxic substances taken during pregnancy, seroconversion of maternal serologies and genetic studies.

A foetal karyotype is recommended for all cases of callosal agenesis, even if they appear to be isolated. In fact, a chromosomal anomaly is detected by karyotype in approximately 5% of these isolated agenesis. The proportion of these chromosomal anomalies detected by foetal karyotype rises to 18% when the ACC is associated with other anomalies (3,46).

Among our patients who had prenatal signs, a foetal karyotype was carried out in only two cases and returned normal.

Chromosomal analysis by DNA chip (ACPA) should be considered when the foetal karyotype returns normal. However, apart from known pathogenic CNVs, the results are more difficult to interpret and the neurological prognosis remains uncertain. Determining whether variants are inherited or *de novo* should also be interpreted with caution, given the variable intra-familial expressivity of ACCs.

2.4. Delivery and birth biometrics

In our series, we noted two cases of prematurity linked to mechanical causes: one case of cervical hernia and one case of hydramnios. Glass et *al* however found a higher risk (x 3.56) of prematurity associated with CCA (9). However, in the sub-group of ACCs with no chromosomal anomalies or syndromes identified, the proportion of premature deliveries was not significantly higher. This suggests that prematurity is related to the presence of other congenital anomalies rather than to callosal agenesis (8).

Congenital microcephaly was found in 40% of our patients and intrauterine growth retardation in 25%. Apart from specific syndromes, biometry at birth was not specified in the various series of ACC reported in the literature.

The high incidence of ACC-associated microcephaly in our series is thought to be related to common pathophysiological mechanisms, in particular abnormalities in the proliferation of neurons and glial cells during brain development. (2).

3. CLINICAL STUDY

3.1 Reason for consultation and referring departments

The majority of our patients were referred by paediatricians and neuropaediatricians, hence the predominance of the following reasons for consultation: developmental delay, intellectual disability and/or cerebral malformation(s).

In the literature, the methods used to recruit VAC cases vary widely from one study to another. This heterogeneity in the populations studied must be taken into account when comparing results.

3.2 Growth

About half of our patients had microcephaly and 15% had macrocephaly. The frequency of microcephaly in reported ACC series varied from 14 to 33%. (47-50)Macrocephaly was rarely specified, with a frequency of 21.7%. (50). Al-Hashim et *al* found only 23% of abnormalities in cranial perimeter (51). This difference with the data in the literature may be linked to different inclusion criteria. In fact, the population in the above-mentioned study were recruited from the radiology department and the discovery of CCA could therefore be fortuitous.

In our series, growth retardation was noted in 37% of cases and advanced staturo-ponderal development in 4% of cases. Apart from specific syndromes, the frequency of association of ACCs with a growth anomaly has not been specified in the literature.

In certain syndromes, ACC is associated with growth retardation, such as Smith-Lemli-Opitz syndrome (OMIM #270400) and Coffin-Siris syndrome (OMIM #135900, 614607, 614608, 614609, 615866, 616938, 617808). (2). Other syndromes combine a staturo-ponderal advance and a CC anomaly, namely Sotos syndrome (OMIM #117550, 617169) (52)Perlman syndrome (OMIM #267000) and Beckwith-Wiedemann syndrome (OMIM #130650) (53). The phenotype of our patients was not suggestive of these syndromes. In these cases, the co-occurrence of two diseases is possible, but only genome-wide studies can confirm or refute this hypothesis.

The short stature associated with obesity in P31 and P32 led us to suggest Borjeson-Forssman-Lehmann syndrome (OMIM #301900) (54).

3.3. Facial dysmorphia

Dysmorphic features were noted in the majority of patients in our series (94%). However, facial dysmorphia was only suggestive of a particular syndrome in about 10% of cases. These were Mowat-Wilson syndrome in P15, orofacial-digital syndrome type 1 in P7 and the syndrome linked to *SPECC1L* missense mutations (Opitz G/BBB type II syndrome) in P9 and P33.

The frequency of facial dysmorphia was high in our study compared with the literature, which ranged from 42 to 73%. (48,51,55,56).

3.4. Anomalies musculoskeletal

Musculoskeletal abnormalities are among the signs most frequently associated with callous agenesis (8). Their frequency in the literature varied from 20% to 37.5% depending on the study (9,47,49,51,56). These abnormalities may be specific and are therefore important in making a diagnosis.

We noted limb anomalies in more than half of our patients [Table I page 20]. However, the majority of these anomalies are considered minor (clinodactyly, camptodactyly) and are not characteristic of a particular syndrome. Only 10% of patients had hexadactyly, an anomaly that is considered characteristic of certain syndromes such as the ciliopathy group. (57). The presence of hexadactyly in four of our patients, together with the other clinical signs, led to the suggestion of a genetic syndrome in three cases: type 1 orofacial-digital syndrome in P7 and Joubert syndrome in P37 and P47.

Other musculoskeletal anomalies were also noted in five patients. The vertebral anomalies found in P43 were, for example, a factor in favour of the suspicion of mosaic trisomy 8 despite a normal karyotype.

3.5. Dermatological abnormalities

Skin and dander abnormalities were found in 17% of our patients. Although the frequency of dermatological abnormalities in ACC is not specified in the literature, several syndromes may associate dermatological involvement with this cerebral malformation. Cockayne's syndrome, for example, is characterised by cutaneous photosensitivity, which is one of the clinical diagnostic criteria for this condition (58).

Dermatoglyphic anomalies were also noted in our series. Among these anomalies, the presence of marked dermatoglyphs with webbing of the fingers reinforced the hypothesis of mosaic trisomy 8 in P43. Indeed, deep palmar and plantar folds are found in 75% of mosaic trisomy 8s (59).

3.6. Abnormalities of the external genitalia

Abnormalities of the external genitalia were present in 19% of our patients and were only found in male patients. This frequency is higher than that reported in the literature (4 to 12.5%) despite a higher sex *ratio* in favour of boys in these series (>1.5) (49,56).

Examination of the external genitalia could reveal an abnormality which would be a key element in the diagnostic orientation. For example, the presence of bilateral cryptorchidism was consistent with Borjeson-Forssman-Lehmann syndrome (OMIM #301900) in P32. The genital anomalies associated with intellectual disability, obesity and short stature were characteristic signs of this syndrome. (54).

3.7. Neurological abnormalities

Consistent with the data in the literature, our study found an unfavourable neurological outcome in patients with syndromic ACC (associated with cerebral or extra-cerebral abnormalities) (4,56). In fact, this unfavourable evolution was noted not only in the populations of syndromic forms but also in those of asymptomatic forms with incidental discovery of ACC on cerebral imaging [Table IX].

Table IX*Frequency of neurological signs in our series and in the literature.*

	Our study	**Romaniello et *al***	**Bedeschi et *al***	**Other studies**
Study population	Genetics department (syndromic ACCs)	Neurorehabilitation Centre (syndromic ACCs)	Patients with ID, learning disabilities and/or epilepsy	Isolated or syndromic ACCs
Engine delay	78%	83%	92%	38 à 78%
Language delay	85%	62%	-	74 à 92%
Hypotonia	59%	-	62%	39 à 77%
Hypertonia/spasticity	41%	-	21%	36%
Intellectual disability	100%	93%	83%	54 %
Epilepsy	41%	41%	35%	39 à 61%
Reference	-	(4)	(56)	(10,48,50,51)

ACC: agenesis of the corpus callosum

Some studies have shown that, among syndromic ACC, those with an identified genetic origin are associated with unfavourable neurological damage (1,56). However, Schell-Apacik et *al* found no significant difference in terms of neurological development according to the presence or absence of an identified genetic anomaly (10).

Furthermore, we found no significant difference in neurological impairment between the different groups: partial *versus* complete agenesis [Table III page 26] or agenesis associated with other encephalic anomalies *versus* isolated [Table VI page 29]. This result is consistent with some studies in the literature, such as that of Goodyear et *al*, although the population studied included children with the incidental discovery of an isolated ACC. (50). Conversely, other studies have found a significant association between the presence of other brain abnormalities and delayed language and/or motor acquisition on the one hand (51)and the presence of these associated anomalies and intellectual disability (4). Furthermore, Romaniello et *al* found a significant difference between the presence of language disorders and the type of CCA (75% in partial agenesis versus 50% in complete agenesis) (4).

Although the neurological consequences of ACC are variable, it appears that the presence of associated encephalic anomalies is probably a major prognostic factor rather than the extent of agenesis (4,51,60,61).

In the literature, epilepsy was found in 35% to 41% of patients with syndromic ACC, which is consistent with our results. The presence or absence of associated encephalic anomalies, particularly cortical anomalies, is associated not only with a higher risk of epileptic disease but also with a higher risk of drug resistance (4,49,51,56). In our series, epilepsy was more frequent in the group of patients with associated encephalic anomalies (50% *versus* 30%) and also in the group with complete agenesis (52% *versus* 24%). However, this difference was not significant. Furthermore, the association between the extent of CCA and the occurrence of epileptic diseases has not been found in the literature (4,56).

3.8. Behavioural problems

Behavioural disorders were noted in 10 of our patients, with eight cases of features of autism spectrum disorder (ASD), one case of polyphagia and one case of behavioural and conduct disorders of the aggressive type. However, it should be noted that these disorders were not systematically identified by a psychologist or psychiatrist.

A recent review of 55 studies reported in the literature on the cognitive and behavioural development associated with ACC showed that 40% of individuals with this cerebral malformation have a deficiency in the social-cognitive domain (recognition of emotions, weakness in the paralinguistic aspects of language and mental abilities). Impaired social cognition can manifest itself in behavioural problems such as autism and attention deficit hyperactivity disorder (62).

These autism spectrum disorders, which are linked to a reduction in the number of interhemispheric connections between the frontal, parietal and occipital cortices, occur in around a third of patients with ACC (63). Thus, it has already been established that CC abnormalities constitute a major risk factor for the development of ASDs with a specificity of associated autistic traits (63). Impaired social interaction occurs later in autistic children with ACC (6 years) compared with autistic children without this malformation (2-3 years) (64). In addition, repetitive and restricted behaviours are less frequent in children with ACC than in other autistic children (65).

Furthermore, in our series we did not find any significant difference in the frequency of these ASD traits between the ACCc and ACCp groups, which is consistent with the data in the literature [Table III page 26]. (63).

3.9. Neurosensory abnormalities

3.9.1. Ophthalmological abnormalities

Sixty-nine per cent of our patients presented with visual disorders, strabismus being the most common anomaly (27%), which is consistent with data in the literature (56). In the literature, we find 20 to 60% of visual anomalies, with no correlation with the type of CCA (10,47,51). Indeed, it has been hypothesised that agenesis of the posterior part of the CC could explain the more frequent occurrence of visual disorders by a defect in the transfer of information between the occipital areas specialised in vision. However, to date no association has been demonstrated (47,51).

In addition, ophthalmological signs can be quite specific and of great help in orienting the diagnosis. For example, ophthalmological involvement has enabled us to distinguish two types of tubulinopathy in our patients: oculomotor paralysis in P24 led us to think of mutations in the *TUBB4A* gene, whereas optic atrophy in P22 led us to think ofTUBB2B (66).

3.9.2 Hearing impairment

Deafness was found in 22% of our patients, whereas in the literature this frequency did not exceed 15%. (10,51). This difference, although not significant, with the data in the literature could be linked to the fact that in our series we only studied syndromic forms, whereas the two aforementioned studies also included isolated forms of ACC.

Apart from these two studies, hearing impairment was not one of the anomalies sought in the other series of ACC reported in the literature. That said, there are genetic syndromes which associate deafness with ACC, such as the Chudley-McCullough syndromes (OMIM #604213) (67)Donnai-Barrow syndrome (OMIM #222448) (68) and Cockayne syndrome (#133540, #216400) (58).

3.10. Other associated congenital malformations

3.10.1. Cardiovascular malformations

Congenital heart disease was identified in 23.5% of our patients. This result is consistent with the literature, where cardiovascular malformations are associated with ACC with a frequency ranging from 13 to 27%. (47,49-51,56).

3.10.2. Urogenital and digestive malformations

Urinary tract malformations are rarely associated with ACCs (2 to 4% in the literature), which is consistent with our results (1 case out of 21). However, the frequency of digestive malformations in our series is lower than that reported in the literature (4% versus 11 to 34%) (50,51) which could be explained by the missing data in our series.

4. CONTRIBUTION OF CEREBRAL MRI IN CORPUS CALLOSUM ANOMALIES

4.1. Agenesis of the corpus callosum: complete or partial

Agenesis of the corpus callosum may be complete (absence of the entire CC) or partial (absence of at least one, but not all, segments of the CC in its anteroposterior axis) [Figure 12].

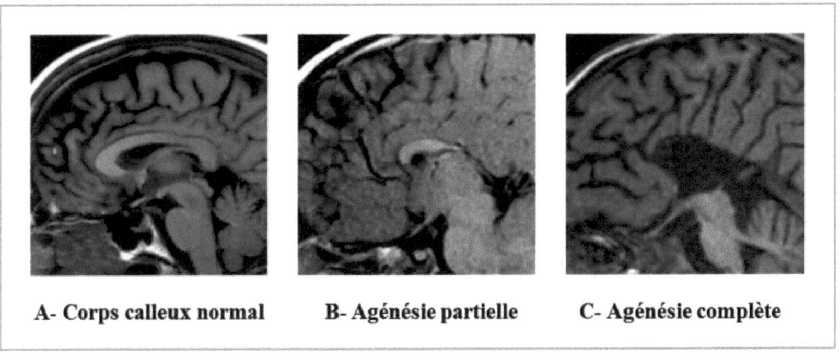

Figure 12*T1-weighted sagittal brain MRI scans (61).*

Complete agenesis was predominant in our series (64%), which is in agreement with the majority of data in the literature, which report 56 to 68% of these complete forms (8,10,50,51). This predominance could be attributed to an easier radiological diagnosis of complete ACCs, to the presence of different classifications of partial anomalies of the CC that can be adopted by radiologists, but also to the ontogeny of the CC (61,69). In fact, in complete forms, the window of action of the factors involved in the onset of callosal agenesis extends throughout the stages of cerebral development, whereas that of partial forms is reduced since the agenesis only occurs at a later stage of development. (5).

Of the partial ACCs in our series, the majority (9/11) were posterior (involving at least the splenium), which is consistent with the data in the literature. This predominance of posterior forms would appear to be related to the chronology of CC development. It develops bidirectionally from the knee, which is the first to individualise (35). However, new studies question this explanation and suggest that posterior agenesis is more likely to result from a dorso-ventral expansion defect of the splenium. These studies suggest that the development of the CC has two origins, one anterior to the knee and one posterior to the splenium (2,21) [Appendix 1: Anatomy of the CC].

The prognosis for complete agenesis is much worse than for partial agenesis. (50). In our series, we found no significant difference in neurological prognosis between these two groups. This difference with the literature is probably related to the fact that the main reason for consultation of our patients was developmental delay.

4.2. Indirect signs of ACC

The diagnosis of ACC on imaging is based not only on the absence of complete or partial agenesis of the CC, but also on the presence of indirect signs.

These signs are divided into anomalies of the lateral ventricles, anomalies of the 3ème ventricle, Probst bands, anomalies of the convolutions and/or anomalies of the other commissures [Table IV page 27]. (70).

In our series, indirect signs were identified in approximately 88% of cases and we found no significant difference in their frequency between the ACCc group (93%) and the ACCp group (80%). However, colpocephaly was identified in the majority of cases in association with complete agenesis in our patients.

In the literature, indirect signs are more constant in complete forms than in partial forms of ACCs, notably Probst's bands, colpocephaly, ascension of the third ventricle and anomalies of the hippocampus (70).

Probst's bands are longitudinal axons of the CC that have failed to cross the midline and therefore form ectopic bundles along the dorsomedial walls of the lateral ventricles. Colpocephaly is due to a reduction in white matter in the occipital cortex leading to expansion of the posterior horns of the lateral ventricles. The third ventricle, the roof of which is normally formed by the corpus callosum, appears to communicate with the interhemispheric scissure and to be high situated in cases of complete absence of the CC (71). Callous agenesis interferes with the development of the hippocampus, leading to trajectory abnormalities and growth defects. In fact, the callosal axons serve as a guide for the development of the other commissures, including the hippocampus (72).

4.3. Brain abnormalities associated with ACC

Agenesis of the corpus callosum was associated with other encephalic anomaly(ies) in 57% of our patients, which is consistent with the literature which reports a frequency ranging from 46 to 83%. (32,51,56).

At least one associated encephalic anomaly was noted in 53% of our patients with ACCc and in 65% of patients with ACCp. This result is consistent with the study by Romaniello et *al*, who found that partial forms were more associated than complete forms with these brain abnormalities (48% *versus* 40%). However, we noted that 66% of the encephalic anomalies were found in patients with complete agenesis, thus showing that these complete forms are often associated with more complex malformations [Table V page 28].

Among the anomalies identified in our patients, anomalies of migration and/or gyration and anomalies of the posterior fossa were the most common (71%), which is consistent with data in the literature (4,10,49,56). These two types of anomaly were predominant in the complete form, which could indicate a common pathophysiological mechanism. (4).

Furthermore, white matter abnormalities were only found in the group of complete agenesis in our patients. Conversely, Neal et *al* found that these anomalies were less frequent in ACCc compared with other CC anomalies. The latter result seems more logical since the callosal axons are established before the onset of myelination, so an abnormality occurring during the myelination process should not contribute to a generalised CC abnormality. (61). This discrepancy with the literature may be related to the limited size of our sample. On the other hand, it has already been reported that cases of complete agenesis are associated with a cholesterol biosynthesis anomaly (desmosterolosis, OMIM #602398) which may be the cause of a white matter anomaly (73). As the clinical picture of our patients is not suggestive of desmosterolosis, this difference with the literature may be related to the limited size of our series.

5. GENETIC STUDY

A genetic cause is identified in 30 to 45% of cases of agenesis of the corpus callosum [Agenesis of the corpus callosum of genetic origin, OMIM #217990]. (10,56). The variability of these genetic causes reflects the complexity of the development of the main inter-hemispheric commissure (2,74). Numerous genes and chromosomal rearrangements have been implicated, with a variety of transmission mechanisms (autosomal dominant, autosomal recessive, X-linked, *de novo* mutation).

5.1. Cytogenetic study

Prenatal or postnatal karyotyping can identify 13 to 17% of the causes of callosal agenesis (8,9). The most frequently identified chromosomal anomalies are trisomy 13, 18, 21 and mosaic trisomy 8 (3). Other aneuploidies have also been reported, namely monosomy of the X chromosome and Klinefelter syndrome (47,XXY) (9,75,76). For these anomalies, the co-occurrence of two pathologies cannot be ruled out (8,75).

In our series, the karyotype was normal in all cases. In P43, despite a normal karyotype, the diagnosis of mosaic trisomy 8 was suggested by the clinical association of suggestive facial dysmorphia, camptodactyly, skeletal malformations, corneal opacity and cerebral malformations. FISH analysis detected mosaic trisomy 8 at a rate of 5%.

In total, only one chromosomal anomaly was identified in our series. This low rate (2%) compared with the literature may be due to our selection criteria. However, in the majority of cases, these chromosomal anomalies are responsible for a polymalformative syndrome diagnosed on prenatal imaging, leading to medical termination of pregnancy or early death *in utero* or after birth.

The use of molecular cytogenetic techniques, more specifically ACPA, has made it possible to identify numerous copy number variations (CNVs) associated with ACC. The identification of these CNVs has made it possible to associate new chromosomal regions (*loci*) and syndromes with ACC and to gain a better understanding of the pathophysiological mechanisms of this cerebral malformation (75).

A recent study assessed the proportion of chromosomal microrearrangements in patients with both corpus callosum anomaly and intellectual disability. Heide et al studied 149 patients using DNA microarrays (SNP illumina). A CNV that was probably or certainly pathogenic was identified in 13% of cases. The most frequently identified rearrangements were inverted duplications with loss of the 8p terminal end (3.2%). Other recurrent CNVs were also identified: deletions 6qter, 18q21, 1q43q44, 17p13.3, 14q12, 3q13, 3p26 and 3q26.

Current recommendations suggest that CAPA should be the first-line examination for ACC associated with intellectual disability (77). We were unable to study the presence or absence of copy number variations in our patients, apart from a single case which came back negative, due to the non-availability of CAPA as a routine test in Tunisia.

5.2 Molecular study

Agenesis of the corpus callosum is genetic in 20 to 35% of cases, and may be monogenic or polygenic. These polygenic ACCs are often isolated and linked to the interaction of numerous modifier genes (1,2).

Metabolic diseases constitute a particular entity among monogenic ACCs. Abnormalities of the CC are often of the hypoplastic type, appearing postnatally and associated with abnormalities of the white matter. The clinical picture often combines developmental delay, recurrent convulsions and metabolic acidosis. Specific dysmorphic features and/or additional congenital anomalies may be associated. ACC is the malformation most frequently found in pyruvate dehydrogenase deficiency (nearly 30% of cases), and is also described in homocystinuria, dopa decarboxylase deficiency and hyperglycaemia without ketosis. (1).

Although ACC is essentially genetic, few genes have been identified to date (75). The use of high-throughput sequencing techniques is making it increasingly possible to identify monogenic causes of ACC, particularly those with no clinical orientation.

Thanks to the sequencing of a panel of 423 genes known to be associated with CC malformations (callosome panel), a recent study has identified a pathogenic mutation in 16% of patients analysed with isolated or associated ACC. The genes involved include *ARID1B* (9% of cases), *ARX*, *MED12*, *FOXG1*, *SPTAN1*, *TUBA1A*, and *ZBTB18*. The identification of a *de novo* mutation in the *ARID1B* gene leading to the appearance of a premature stop codon was one of the major results of this study. *ARID1B* encodes a subunit of the SWI/SNF complex which plays a crucial role in the expression of target genes during development. Mutations in this gene are known to be involved in Coffin-Siris syndrome (OMIM #135900), which is characterised by constant ID, IUGR, mild dysmorphia and hypo/aplasia of the nails and third phalanges predominating in the fifth fingers and toes. An anomaly of the CC (agenesis, dysgenesis or hypoplasia) was found in about half the cases. Most of the patients in the above-mentioned cohort with an *ARID1B* mutation had a phenotype compatible with Coffin-Siris syndrome, but none of them had abnormalities of the phalanges and toes, which explains why this diagnosis was not made in all patients. *ARID1B* mutations are currently known to be the major cause of corpus callosum anomalies associated with intellectual disability (78,79). In the same study, exome sequencing of callosome-negative cases identified a likely pathogenic mutation in 30% of patients, and proposed the analysis of new candidate genes for the other cases without an established diagnosis.

This study illustrates the value of high-throughput sequencing in the diagnosis of isolated ACCs or ACCs without diagnostic orientation, but also in the identification of new monogenic causes and new syndromes that may be associated with callosal agenesis.

6. DIAGNOSTIC ORIENTATION

6.1. Causes of ACCs

Although CCA is essentially genetic, 55-70% of the aetiologies of callosal agenesis cannot be identified by clinical assessment (10,56). These cases of CCA for which there is no diagnostic orientation make the interpretation of genetic analyses difficult (10,75).

Furthermore, the aetiology of ACC is not genetic in a proportion of these patients. In fact, callosal agenesis is linked not only to genetic factors but also to environmental factors, namely infectious, toxic and ischaemic causes (1-3) [Table X].

Table X*Causes of agenesis of the corpus callosum (ACC).*

Causes	Subtype	Additional notes	Reference
Genetics	Anomalies chromosomal	Chromosomal abnormalities are identified by karyotype in 13 to 17% of ACCs.	(4,8,9)
	Copy number variations (CNV): loss or gain	*De novo* CNVs detected by DNA chips are identified in 13% of cases postnatally.	(77)

	Monogenic diseases (autosomal or X-linked, Mendelian or *de novo* transmission)	A monogenic cause is identified in 20 to 35% of syndromic ACCs. Metabolic causes are a special case.	(10,56)
	Polygenic diseases	This could explain many cases of ACC with no identifiable cause, particularly isolated agenesis.	(2,21)
Environmental	Antenatal exposure to toxic substances	The best-known example is alcohol. - Maternal phenylketonuria: Rare (especially since neonatal screening was introduced in many countries in the 1960s)	(1,2,6,7)
	Antenatal infections	- Examples: cytomegalovirus, toxoplasmosis, rubella and influenza. - Often with other associated anomalies.	
	Hypoxic/vascular causes	Rare	

Foetal alcohol syndrome is a typical example of the toxic causes of ACCs (described in detail in the chapter entitled "Special features of pregnancy" on page 40).

Among infectious causes, congenital toxoplasmosis, congenital CMV infection and congenital rubella are inconsistently associated with ACC.

The anoxo-ischaemic cause in the pre- or peri-natal period is reported in premature babies. CCAs have been described in these patients, notably posterior agenesis of the CC, associated with lesions of periventricular leukomalacia (80).

6.2. Penetration of syndromic ACCs

More than 200 syndromes with an identified genetic cause, listed in the OMIM database, are more or less consistently associated with ACC (2,3).

The genetic syndromes consistently associated with ACC are presented in table XI.

Other syndromes with no identified genetic cause are also constantly associated with callous agenesis, namely Aicardi syndrome (OMIM #304050), which is characterised by a triad associating CCA, infantile spasms and chorioretinal lacunae. It is probably linked to de novo mutations on chromosome X (81,82).

Table XI*Genetic syndromes consistently associated with agenesis of the corpus callosum (2).*

Syndromes	OMIM	Gene(s)	Heredity	Other characteristic signs	Reference (1[er] author)
ACC-DI-coloboma-micrognathia syndrome	300472	*IGBP1* (Xq13.1)	XLR	Coloboma of the iris or optic nerve, DI	Graham 2003 (83)
Chudley-McCullough syndrome	604213	*GPSM2* (1p13.3)	AR	Deafness, interhemispheric cyst, cerebral/cerebellar dyspalsy	Doherty 2012 (84)
Acro-calcific syndrome	200990	*KIF7* (15q26.1) *Gli3* (7p14.1)	AR	Polydactyly, MDW, DI	Ibisler 2015 (85) Putoux 2018 (86)
Hydrolethalus syndrome	236680	*HYLS1* (11q24.2)	AR	Hydrocephalus, thalamic	Paetau 2008 (87)

	614120	*KIF7* (15q26.1)		fusion, gyration anomalies	Putoux 2011 (88)
ACC-genital anomalies syndrome (Proud syndrome)	300004	*ARX* (Xp21.3)	XLR	DI, genital deformities, limb contractures, scoliosis	Kato 2004 (89)
Polymicrogyria	610031	*TUBB2B* (6p25.2)	AD	Asymmetric polymicrogyria, cerebellar hypoplasia	Jaglin 2009 (90)
Andermann syndrome	218000	*SLC12A6* (15q14)	AR	Peripheral neuropathy	Howard 2002 (91) Bowerman 2017 (92)
Desmosterolosis	602398	*DHCR24* (1p32.3)	AR	High cholesterol, DF	Schaaf 2011 (93)
Cerebellopontine hypoplasia type 9	615809	*AMPD2* (1p13.3)	AR	Pontocerebellar hypoplasia	Kortüm 2018 (94)
Vici syndrome	242840	*EPG5* (18q12.3-q21.1)	AR	Growth retardation, hypopigmentation	Maillard 2017 (95)

AD: autosomal dominant, **ACC**: agenesis of the corpus callosum, **AR**: autosomal recessive, **DF**: facial dysmorphia, **ID**: intellectual disability, **FP**: cleft palate, **MDW**: Dandy-Walker malformation, **XLR**: X-linked recessive.

ACC is also frequently but not consistently found in certain syndromes such as: Donnai-Barrow syndrome (almost all cases of (96)), Meckel syndrome (57%), Mowat-Wilson syndrome (43%), oro-facio-digital syndrome type 1 (81%), microdeletion 1q42-q44 syndrome (80%) and rearrangements of the short arm of chromosome 8 (66% in mosaic tetrasomies 8p). (2).

Among the syndromes and genetic anomalies identified in our series, type 1 orofacial-digital syndrome, Mowat-Wilson syndrome, Opitz syndrome and mosaic trisomy 8 are classically described in association with ACC [Table XII].

The variability in the penetrance of this cerebral malformation highlights the involvement of other genetic and environmental factors in the ontogeny of ACC.

Table XII*Genetic syndromes mentioned in our patients.*

Syndrome (OMIM)	**Heredity**	**Majority gene(s) (*Locus*)**	**Frequent signs**	**CNS abnormalities**	**Reference (1er author)**
Cockayne syndrome (#133540, #216400)	AR	*ERCC6* (10q11.23) and *ERCC8* (5q12.1)	- Delayed development - Progressive RC and microcephaly - Major lipoatrophy - Skin photosensitivity, deafness - Pigmentary retinopathy and/or cataracts - Enamel hypoplasia	CNS abnormalities 83.5% : - Calcifications 55 - SB anomalies 38 - Atrophy - CC abnormalities: hypoplasia or atrophy (knee, splenium)	- Laugel 2013 (58) - Koob 2016 (97) - Wilson 2016 (98)

Oro-Facio-Digital syndrome type 1 (OFD1; #311200)	XLD	*OFD1* (Xp22.2) (SNV or CNV)	- Oral anomalies 95% (tongue, enamel and teeth) - DF 82.8 - Limb abnormalities 88 - Mild to moderate ID 46.1% - Cystic diseases	CNS abnormality 50% : - CC abnormalities 81.2% (ACCc) - Interhemispheric cysts - Vermian hypoplasia - Gyration abnormalities	- Bisschoff 2013 (99) - Bruel 2017 (100)
Joubert syndrome	AR XLR	>30 primary cilium genes *OFD1* (Xp22.2)	- Developmental delay and ID - Respiratory problems - Cerebellar ataxia - Ocular anomalies: Oculomotor apraxia 80%,	- Molar tooth sign with hypoplasia or vermian agenesis 100%.	- Poretti 2017 (101) - Wang 2018 (102) - Fleming 2017 (103)

			strabismus 74%, nystagmus 72%, retinal dystrophy - Kidney 30% and heart abnormalities - Polydactyly	- Posterior fossa enlarged in 42%, with appearance similar to MDW - Malrotation of seahorses 28 - Ventriculomegaly 23 - Agenesis or dysgenesis of the CC 9	- Karp 2012 (104)
***SPECC1L* syndrome (**Opitz G/BBB type II syndrome**)** (#145410)	AD (*de novo* or familial cases)	*SPECC1L* missense mutations (22q11.23)	- DF: hypertelorism, FP oblique downwards and outwards, palpebral ptosis, wide bridge of nose, anteverted	CNS abnormality 67% : - CC anomalies	Bhoj 2018 (105)

			nostrils, long philtrum, micrognathia - Omphalocele, umbilical hernia - Bicornuate uterus - Delayed development 61	- Ventriculomegaly	
Mowat-Wilson syndrome (#235730)	AD *de novo*	ZEB2 (2q22.3) (truncating or missense mutations)	- Characteristic DF: high forehead, thick eyebrows thinned in the middle, hypertelorism, large deep-set eyes, broad bridge of nose with round tip and prominent columella, open mouth, M-shaped upper lip, prominent triangular chin, anteverted earlobes with or without central depression.	CNS abnormality 96% : - CC anomalies 79.6% (complete or partial agenesis, hypoplasia) - Hippocampal abnormalities 77.8	- Garavelli 2017 (106) - Ivanovski 2018 (107)

			- Moderate to severe ID and epilepsy 78 - Microcephaly 78% and short stature 46%. - Hirschsprung's disease 44 - Genital anomalies (hypospadias 60%, cryptorchidism 41%) and cardiovascular anomalies 58%.	- Dilatation of lateral ventricles 68.5 - SB abnormalities	
Serine deficiency	AR	*PHGDH* (1p12) or *PSPH* (7p11.2)	- Congenital microcephaly and IUGR - Bilateral congenital cataract -Spastic tetraplegia and epilepsy - Delayed development	- Lissencephaly 50% - CC anomalies 33%: agenesis or hypoplasia	- El-Hattab 2016 (108) - Darouich 2016 (109)

				- Hypoplasia of the cerebellum 40 - MDW	
Tubulinopathies (#610031) (*#612438*)	AD or AR	Gene heterogeneity	- Congenital microcephaly - Epilepsy - Ophthalmological abnormalities	Anomalies in cortical and commissural development	Romaniello 2018 and 2015 (66,110)
	AD	*TUBB2B* (6p25.2)	- Often severe developmental delay - Optic atrophy, strabismus, palpebral ptosis	- Perisylvian or central region polymicrogyria - Agenesis or hypoplasia of the CC	
	AD *De novo*	*TUBB4A* (19p13.3)	- Progressive developmental delay	- Leukodystrophy	

			- Small size - Dystonia, spasticity - Oculomotor paralysis, nystagmus	- Hypomyelination - Atrophy of the basal ganglia - CC anomalies	
Borjeson-Forssman-Lehmann syndrome (#301900)	XLR	*PHF6* (Xq26.2)	- Neonatal hypotonia - Mild to severe ID, behavioural problems - DF: protruding orbital arches, enophthalmos, palpebral ptosis - Obesity 75%, short stature - Genital anomalies, gynaecomastia in adolescence	- Gyration abnormalities - Heterotopia - Ventriculomegaly - CC anomalies: agenesis or hypoplasia	- Jahani-Asl 2016 (54) - Birrell 2003 (111)
Seckel syndrome	AR	Genetic heterogeneity	- Prenatal proportional dwarfism	Rare CNS malformations :	- Shanske 1997 (112)

			- Bird's head DF: beaked nose, receding forehead, prominent eyes and micrognathia. - DI often mild to moderate, severe if associated with CNS malformations	- CC anomalies: hypoplasia or agenesis - Simplification of *gyri* - Migration abnormalities	-Faivre 2002 (113) - Verloes 1993 (114)
15q24 microdeletion syndrome	*De novo* (1.7 to 6.1 Mb)	Minimal region *CYP11A1*, *SEMA7A*, *CPLX3*, *ARID3B*, *STRA6*, *SIN3A* and *CSK*	- Hypotonia, mild to severe ID - DF: high forehead, hypertelorism, epicanthus, FP oblique downwards and outwards, wide depressed nasal root, long effaced philtrum, ear anomalies - Growth retardation	MRI abnormalities 44 - CC anomalies - Cortical atrophy - Focal dysplasia	Magoulas and El-Hattab 2012 (115)

		- Skeletal, genital and ocular abnormalities -Behavioural problems	- Hypoplasia of the olfactory bulbs	
Mosaic of Trisomy 8	*De novo*	- Mild to severe ID - DF, growth retardation - Skeletal (vertebral++), cardiovascular and urinary tract anomalies - Deep palmar and plantar folds (75%) -Corneal opacities and strabismus	- ACC	Giraldo 2016 (59)

(AD: autosomal dominant, AR: autosomal recessive, ACC: agenesis of the corpus callosum, CNV: copy number variation, DF: facial dysmorphia, FP: cleft palate, MDW: Dandy-Walker malformation, CNS: central nervous system, SNV: *single nucleotide variation*, XLD: X-linked dominant, XLR: X-linked recessive).

6.3. Pathophysiological mechanisms of ACCs

The various factors associated with callosal agenesis occur at different stages of brain development, making it possible to classify ACCs into five groups (2,7) :

6.3.1. Abnormalities in glial and/or neuronal proliferation

Many of the molecules involved in glial and/or neuronal proliferation often play a major role in development. Consequently, CC anomalies resulting from dysfunction of these molecules are never isolated and are part of syndromic ACCs. In this group, callosal agenesis is often associated with microcephaly and cortical disorganisation. The presence of these cortical anomalies makes it possible to differentiate this group from primary microcephalias of autosomal recessive transmission. (2).

Among the genetic syndromes included in this group, we mentioned Seckel, Cockayne, Mowat-Wilson and Borjeson-Forssman-Lehmann syndromes in our patients. The respective genes in these syndromes, *SCKL* (*1*, *2* or *4 to 10*), *ERCC* (in particular *6* and *8*), *ZEB2* and *PHF6* code for transcription factors and therefore regulate the expression of other genes involved in cell proliferation.

In Mowat-Wilson syndrome, the callous phenotype varies within the same family. This variable penetrance of ACC could be explained by the presence of modifier genes (116).

6.3.2. Abnormalities in the formation or recognition of the midline

Defects in the invagination of the dorsal prosencephalon lead to the formation of a single hollow vesicle (holoprosencephaly), with consequent loss of all medial structures, including the corpus callosum. This condition may affect the whole of the telencephalon, or may be limited to the caudal or rostral regions. In the latter case, the CC may form in part, resulting in hypoplasia or partial agenesis. In fact, this defect in diverticulation of the telencephalon is thought to be responsible for the loss of a substrate by which the callosal axons can cross the median line (117). This substrate is the guidance molecules secreted by the glial cells of the median line to define the migration trajectories of commissural axons.

Among the syndromes included in this group, we identified Joubert syndrome in three of our patients. This syndrome, linked to dysfunction of the primary cilium (ciliopathy), may be due to a defect in the expression of KIF7. This protein plays a central role in the *Sonic Hedgehog* (SHH) signalling pathway by maintaining the balance between the repressive (GLI3R) and activating (GLI3A) forms of the GLI3 protein, a major transcription factor in this pathway. Mutations in *KIF7* lead to a reduction in GLI3R and overexpression of the target genes of the SHH pathway. The SHH pathway plays a role in the ventral regionalisation of the neural tube and is expressed by the notochord, the basal plate of the neural tube and the prechordal plate. These structures interact with the overlying ectoderm to establish the midline. Haploinsufficiency of SHH in humans is one of the major causes of holoprosencephaly.

ACC is part of the phenotypic spectrum of several other ciliopathies which share an alteration in the SHH pathway, in particular acro-callous, hydrolethalus and Meckel syndromes in which callosal agenesis is a frequent sign. (2).

In addition, orofacial-digital syndrome type 1, identified in one of our patients, is also classified in this group of midline anomalies. This syndrome is due to mutations in the *OFD1* gene, which codes for a protein located in the centrosome and basal body of primary cilia.

6.3.3. Abnormalities in callosal neuron migration and specialisation

This group of diseases is linked to mutations in genes involved either in the structure of microtubules (tubulins) or in their stabilisation (*DCX*, *DCLK1*). The phenotype is often severe, combining ACC with lissencephaly and nodular heterotopia. Among the syndromes mentioned in our patients are tubulinopathies in which callosal agenesis is linked to an abnormality in neuronal migration.

In addition, the syndrome linked to *SPECC1L* mutations in two of our patients could be classified in this group. This gene codes for a protein containing a *coiled-coil* domain that ensures its dimerisation, which may play a critical role in the organisation of the actin cytoskeleton (www.genecards.org).

6.3.4. Axonal guidance abnormalities

Rare cases of CCA in association with this abnormality of brain development have been reported, with the exception of cranio-fronto-nasal syndrome (OMIM #304110), which may be linked to mutations in the *EFNB1* gene. This gene codes for the ephrin-B1 protein, which is expressed by glial cells. Glial cells help to define the migratory trajectories of callosal axons. (2).

6.3.5. Synaptogenesis abnormalities

Several enzyme deficiencies are included in this group and are associated with hypoplasia of the CC rather than agenesis, which could be linked either to a defect in the postnatal development of the central nervous system or to an anomaly of the white matter. Examples of these aetiologies include pyruvate dehydrogenase deficiency and serine deficiency. (2). The latter was mentioned in one of our patients and is linked to a deficiency of one of the enzymes in the L-serine biosynthesis pathway: phosphoglycerate dehydrogenase (PGDH), phosphoserine aminotransferase (PSAT) or phosphoserine phosphatase (PSP) (108). L-serine is an amino acid expressed specifically in astrocytes where it is the precursor of D-serine, the main co-agonist of postsynaptic NMDAR receptors (*N-methyl-d-aspartate receptor*) which are necessary for synaptic activity and plasticity. (118).

Desmosterolosis (3-beta-hydroxysterol-delta24-reductase deficiency) and Smith-Lemli-Opitz syndrome (7-dehydrocholesterol reductase deficiency) are other enzyme deficiencies which may be associated with a CC anomaly and which have been classified in this group. (2). However, these two diseases are linked to a deficit in the synthesis of cholesterol, which is required not only for myelination but also for post-translational modifications of the SHH morphogen (119). Consequently, the ACC associated with these two enzyme deficiencies could be linked to a midline anomaly. (2).

7. GENETIC COUNCIL

7.1. Prenatal genetic counselling

Genetic counselling depends mainly on whether or not an aetiological diagnosis has been made.

When an aetiology is determined, it is very often a syndromic form of callosal agenesis. Numerous studies have shown that the prognosis for CCA is poorer when it is associated with other cerebral or extra-cerebral malformations, and couples may consider medical termination of pregnancy (IMG) in the case of callosal agenesis discovered antenatally (4,8). CCA may thus give rise to a request for a termination of pregnancy because the unborn child is likely to suffer from a particularly serious condition under article 214 of the Tunisian Penal Code.

When the aetiological investigation is negative, and in the absence of poor prognostic factors (associated cerebral or extra-cerebral malformations), CC agenesis is considered to be isolated. These isolated forms have a more uncertain prognosis, with some forms being asymptomatic and others associated with developmental disorders of varying severity. (120). Although the prognosis for isolated ACCs is therefore generally more favourable, it remains uncertain and makes prenatal advice tricky. It remains difficult for the geneticist to reassure couples when the malformation appears isolated prenatally, firstly because it may be associated with other malformations discovered after birth and secondly because isolated ACC is often accompanied by cognitive difficulties whose impact on the child's autonomy and integration is difficult to predict. (120). There is no consensus on whether or not to continue the pregnancy in apparently isolated CCAs. In our series, given the isolated nature of the cerebral anomalies discovered antenatally, no termination of pregnancy was proposed.

7.2. Postnatal genetic counselling

By identifying the genetic causes of ACC, couples can be offered appropriate genetic counselling, both in terms of prognosis and risk of recurrence.

When a syndrome is evoked clinically, a risk of recurrence, based on the mode of transmission of this pathology, could be explained to the couple even in the absence of genetic confirmation. However, given the intra-familial heterogeneity, the prognosis remains uncertain.

Despite the presence of a diagnostic referral in around 40% of our patients, no genetic confirmation was carried out. Prenatal molecular diagnosis could not therefore be proposed, and only ultrasound monitoring by a specialist doctor was recommended, even for cases with a low risk of recurrence.

Apart from ultrasound monitoring, the risk of recurrence cannot be estimated for cases of callosal agenesis without diagnostic guidance.

The consequences of CCA are therefore often difficult to establish with certainty, and sometimes only the child's follow-up will enable us to assess the true extent and severity of the condition. Early and prolonged developmental monitoring of these children is essential in order to provide appropriate care for each child, and to improve our knowledge of this malformation with a view to adapting the genetic counselling given to couples in the prenatal period.

Conclusion

CONCLUSION

Agenesis of the corpus callosum (ACC) is the most common cerebral malformation. It corresponds to a complete or partial absence of formation of this main interhemispheric commissure.

ACC may be isolated or associated with other malformations (cerebral or extra-cerebral malformations). Its clinical expression varies from asymptomatic forms, where ACC is discovered by chance, to syndromic forms with severe intellectual disability.

Callous agenesis, both isolated and syndromic, is highly heterogeneous from a genetic point of view, and is part of a known syndrome in around a third of cases. A genetic cause is identified in 30 to 45% of cases.

The aims of our work were to determine the epidemiological and clinical characteristics of syndromic agenesis of the corpus callosum, and to emphasise the importance of clinical examination in the aetiological orientation of these ACCs.

By comparing our results with the data in the literature, we were able to make the following observations:

Epidemiological data:

- The age of the patients at the first consultation was young, explained by the fact that the patients included in our study have syndromic ACC, as asymptomatic forms with fortuitous and late discovery of ACC on brain imaging are not recruited in our department.
- The majority of our patients were from the north of Tunisia, which is explained by a recruitment bias.
- Consanguinity was noted in 38% of cases and is thought to be a risk factor for ACC, which is part of the autosomal recessive inheritance syndromes.

- The average maternal age at conception was slightly higher than the average age of parturients in Tunisia, in line with the literature, and is thought to be linked to the higher risk of chromosomal abnormalities, which is correlated with maternal age.

In terms of prenatal diagnosis, prenatal signs were found at the second-trimester ultrasound in only 16% of cases. This low rate compared with that reported in the literature (60-90%), could be explained by the fact that the second-trimester ultrasound was not systematically performed by a doctor specialising in foetal imaging. Among our patients who had prenatal signs, a foetal karyotype, which should be systematically indicated, was carried out in only two cases and came back normal.

Clinical data:

- The majority of our patients were referred for developmental delay, intellectual disability and/or cerebral malformation(s).

- The most frequent signs revealed by the clinical examination were: microcephaly, which was more frequent in our series than in the literature; growth retardation; facial dysmorphia, which was almost constant but was only suggestive of a particular syndrome in about 10% of cases; musculoskeletal anomalies, particularly of the limbs; and anomalies of the external genitalia, which were only found in male patients. Sixty-nine per cent of patients had visual problems and 22% were deaf. Congenital heart disease was identified in 23.5% of cases.

- Consistent with the literature, our study found an unfavourable neurological outcome in patients with syndromic ACC (associated with cerebral or extra-cerebral abnormalities). We noted delayed motor acquisition in 78% of cases, delayed language in 85% of cases, constant intellectual disability in patients aged over three years and epilepsy in 41% of cases.

- Behavioural problems were noted in 10 patients, with a predominance of autism spectrum disorder features.

Regarding brain MRI data:

- Consistent with the literature, complete agenesis was predominant in our series and most partial forms were posterior.
- In our series, indirect signs were identified in approximately 88% of cases, with no significant difference between complete and partial forms, whereas in the literature these signs are more associated with complete agenesis.
- Callous agenesis was associated with other encephalic anomaly(ies) in 57% of cases, with a predominance of cortical and/or neuronal migration anomalies and posterior fossa anomalies, which is consistent with data in the literature. The presence of these cerebral malformations is a poor prognostic factor for the neurocognitive development of children with ACC.

In terms of aetiological diagnosis, cytogenetic techniques identified a chromosomal anomaly in one patient (mosaic trisomy 8). Targeted molecular studies were normal. High-throughput sequencing was not performed in any patient, as it is not available as a routine diagnostic procedure in Tunisia.

Thanks to the clinical study of each patient, we were able to orientate the diagnosis in more than 37% (16/43) of families and provide appropriate genetic counselling despite the absence of cytogenetic or molecular confirmation.

Finally, we plan to supplement this work with an etiological study using molecular cytogenetic (ACPA) and molecular biology (targeted or high throughput sequencing) techniques in our patients with a view to :

- Search for a genotype-phenotype correlation in the patients studied.
- Provide couples with appropriate genetic counselling and offer them prenatal diagnosis to prevent recurrence of this anomaly in familial forms.

- Identify new genetic causes, chromosomal anomalies or genetic causes, of agenesis of the corpus callosum without diagnostic orientation.

Bibliography

BIBLIOGRAPHY

1. Palmer EE, Mowat D. Agenesis of the corpus callosum: a clinical approach to diagnosis. Am J Med Genet C Semin Med Genet. June 2014;166C(2):184-97.

2. Edwards TJ, Sherr EH, Barkovich AJ, Richards LJ. Clinical, genetic and imaging findings identify new causes for corpus callosum development syndromes. Brain J Neurol. June 2014;137(Pt 6):1579-613.

3. Leombroni M, Khalil A, Liberati M, D'Antonio F. Fetal midline anomalies: Diagnosis and counselling Part 1: Corpus callosum anomalies. Eur J Paediatr Neurol EJPN Off J Eur Paediatr Neurol Soc. nov 2018;22(6):951-62.

4. Romaniello R, Marelli S, Giorda R, Bedeschi MF, Bonaglia MC, Arrigoni F, et al. Clinical Characterization, Genetics, and Long-Term Follow-up of a Large Cohort of Patients With Agenesis of the Corpus Callosum. J Child Neurol. 2017;32(1):60-71.

5. Folliot-Le Doussal L, Chadie A, Brasseur-Daudruy M, Verspyck E, Saugier-Veber P, Marret S, et al. Neurodevelopmental outcome in prenatally diagnosed isolated agenesis of the corpus callosum. Early Hum Dev. 2018;116:9-16.

6. des Portes V, Rolland A, Velazquez-Dominguez J, Peyric E, Cordier M-P, Gaucherand P, et al. Outcome of isolated agenesis of the corpus callosum: A population-based prospective study. Eur J Paediatr Neurol EJPN Off J Eur Paediatr Neurol Soc. Jan 2018;22(1):82-92.

7. Paul LK, Brown WS, Adolphs R, Tyszka JM, Richards LJ, Mukherjee P, et al. Agenesis of the corpus callosum: genetic, developmental and functional aspects of connectivity. Nat Rev Neurosci. Apr 2007;8(4):287-99.

8. Ballardini E, Marino P, Maietti E, Astolfi G, Neville AJ. Prevalence and associated factors for agenesis of corpus callosum in Emilia Romagna (1981-2015). Eur J Med Genet. Sep 2018;61(9):524-30.

9. Glass HC, Shaw GM, Ma C, Sherr EH. Agenesis of the Corpus Callosum in California 1983-2003: A Population-Based Study. Am J Med Genet A. 2008 Oct 1;146A(19):2495-500.

10. Schell-Apacik CC, Wagner K, Bihler M, Ertl-Wagner B, Heinrich U, Klopocki E, et al. Agenesis and dysgenesis of the corpus callosum: clinical, genetic and neuroimaging findings in a series of 41 patients. Am J Med Genet A. 1 Oct 2008;146A(19):2501-11.

11. Ben Halim N, Ben Alaya Bouafif N, Romdhane L, Kefi Ben Atig R, Chouchane I, Bouyacoub Y, et al. Consanguinity, endogamy, and genetic disorders in Tunisia. J Community Genet. Apr 2013;4(2):273-84.

12. Sztriha L. Spectrum of corpus callosum agenesis. Pediatr Neurol. Feb 2005;32(2):94-101.

13. Al-Gazali L, Hamamy H. Consanguinity and dysmorphology in Arabs. Hum Hered. 2014;77(1-4):93-107.

14. Bittles AH. Consanguineous marriage and childhood health. Dev Med Child Neurol. August 2003;45(8):571-6.

15. Ben Halim N, Hsouna S, Lasram K, Rejeb I, Walha A, Talmoudi F, et al. Differential impact of consanguineous marriages on autosomal recessive diseases in Tunisia. Am J Hum Biol Off J Hum Biol Counc. Apr 2016;28(2):171-80.

16. El Mhamdi S, Ben Salem K, Bouanene I, Soussi Soltani M. [Chronological observation of the epidemiological characteristics of perinatal indicators in the Monastir health region (Tunisia) between 1994 and 2008]. Sante Publique Vandoeuvre--Nancy Fr. August 2011;23(4):287-95.

17. Zhang X-H, Qiu L-Q, Ye Y-H, Xu J. Chromosomal abnormalities: subgroup analysis by maternal age and perinatal features in zhejiang province of China, 2011-2015. Ital J Pediatr. may 2017;43:47.

18. Kim YJ, Lee JE, Kim SH, Shim SS, Cha DH. Maternal age-specific rates of fetal chromosomal abnormalities in Korean pregnant women of advanced maternal age. Obstet Gynecol Sci. May 2013;56(3):160-6.

19. Hunter N. Meiotic Recombination: The Essence of Heredity. Cold Spring Harb Perspect Biol.Dec 2017;7(12):a016618.

20. Riley EP, Mattson SN, Sowell ER, Jernigan TL, Sobel DF, Jones KL. Abnormalities of the corpus callosum in children prenatally exposed to alcohol. Alcohol Clin Exp Res. Oct 1995;19(5):1198-202.

21. Paul LK. Developmental malformation of the corpus callosum: a review of typical callosal development and examples of developmental disorders with callosal involvement. J Neurodev Disord. March 2011;3(1):3-27.

22. Bookstein FL, Sampson PD, Connor PD, Streissguth AP. Midline corpus callosum is a neuroanatomical focus of fetal alcohol damage. Anat Rec. June 15, 2002;269(3):162-74.

23. Caputo C, Wood E, Jabbour L. Impact of fetal alcohol exposure on body systems: A systematic review. Birth Defects Res Part C Embryo Today Rev. June 2016;108(2):174-80.

24. Kiecker C. The chick embryo as a model for the effects of prenatal exposure to alcohol on craniofacial development. Dev Biol. 15 2016;415(2):314-25.

25. Kietzman HW, Everson JL, Sulik KK, Lipinski RJ. The teratogenic effects of prenatal ethanol exposure are exacerbated by Sonic Hedgehog or GLI2 haploinsufficiency in the mouse. PloS One. 2014;9(2):e89448.

26. Denny L, Coles S, Blitz R. Fetal Alcohol Syndrome and Fetal Alcohol Spectrum Disorders. Am Fam Physician. 15 Oct 2017;96(8):515-22.

27. Vallée L, Cuvellier JC. Foetal alcohol syndrome: central nervous system lesions and clinical phenotype. Pathol Biol (Paris). Nov 2001;49(9):732-7.

28. Yu R, Deochand C, Krotow A, Leão R, Tong M, Agarwal AR, et al. Tobacco Smoke-Induced Brain White Matter Myelin Dysfunction: Potential Co-Factor Role of Smoking in Neurodegeneration. J Alzheimers Dis JAD. 2016;50(1):133-48.

29. Umene-Nakano W, Yoshimura R, Kakeda S, Watanabe K, Hayashi K, Nishimura J, et al. Abnormal white matter integrity in the corpus callosum among smokers: tract-based spatial statistics. PloS One. 2014;9(2):e87890.

30. Hudkins M, O'Neill J, Tobias MC, Bartzokis G, London ED. Cigarette smoking and white matter microstructure. Psychopharmacology (Berl). May 2012;221(2):285-95.

31. Assistance médicale à la procréation (AMP) [Internet]. Inserm - Science for health. [cited 11 Apr 2019]. Available from: https://www.inserm.fr/information-en-sante/dossiers-information/assistance-medicale-procreation-amp

32. Volpe P, Paladini D, Resta M, Stanziano A, Salvatore M, Quarantelli M, et al. Characteristics, associations and outcome of partial agenesis of the corpus callosum in the fetus. Ultrasound Obstet Gynecol Off J Int Soc Ultrasound Obstet Gynecol. May 2006;27(5):509-16.

33. Richards LJ, Plachez C, Ren T. Mechanisms regulating the development of the corpus callosum and its agenesis in mouse and human. Clin Genet. Oct 2004;66(4):276-89.

34. Tanaka-Arakawa MM, Matsui M, Tanaka C, Uematsu A, Uda S, Miura K, et al. Developmental changes in the corpus callosum from infancy to early adulthood: a structural magnetic resonance imaging study. PloS One. 2015;10(3):e0118760.

35. Paulet E, Delorme B, Loisiel D, Lepinard C, Triau S, Boussion F, et al. Place de l'IRM fœtale dans la prise en charge des agénésies du corps calleux. Feuillets de Radiologie.oct 2005;45(5):363-371.

36. De Keersmaecker B, Pottel H, Naulaers G, De Catte L. Sonographic Development of the Pericallosal Vascularization in the First and Early Second Trimester of Pregnancy. AJNR Am J Neuroradiol. 2018;39(3):589-96.

37. Pilu G, Sandri F, Perolo A, Pittalis MC, Grisolia G, Cocchi G, et al. Sonography of fetal agenesis of the corpus callosum: a survey of 35 cases. Ultrasound Obstet Gynecol Off J Int Soc Ultrasound Obstet Gynecol. 1 Sept 1993;3(5):318-29.

38. Pashaj S, Merz E. Detection of Fetal Corpus Callosum Abnormalities by Means of 3D Ultrasound. Ultraschall Med Stuttg Ger 1980. Apr 2016;37(2):185-94.

39. Karl K, Esser T, Heling KS, Chaoui R. Cavum septi pellucidi (CSP) ratio: a marker for partial agenesis of the fetal corpus callosum. Ultrasound Obstet Gynecol Off J Int Soc Ultrasound Obstet Gynecol. sept 2017;50(3):336-41.

40 Zhao D, Wang B, Cai A. Utility of indirect sonographic signs (including cavum septum pellucidum ratio) in midgestational screening for partial agenesis of corpus callosum. J Clin Ultrasound JCU. March 5, 2019; 1-5.

41. Jarre A, Llorens Salvador R, Montoliu Fornas G, Montoya Filardi A. Value of brain MRI when sonography raises suspicion of agenesis of the corpus callosum in fetuses. Radiologia. June 2017;59(3):226-31.

42. Fratelli N, Papageorghiou AT, Prefumo F, Bakalis S, Homfray T, Thilaganathan B. Outcome of prenatally diagnosed agenesis of the corpus callosum. Prenat Diagn. June 2007;27(6):512-7.

43. Manevich-Mazor M, Weissmann-Brenner A, Bar Yosef O, Hoffmann C, Mazor RD, Mosheva M, et al. Added Value of Fetal MRI in the Evaluation of Fetal Anomalies of the Corpus Callosum: A Retrospective Analysis of 78 Cases. Ultraschall Med Stuttg Ger 1980. 2018;39(5):513-25.

44. Falip C, Hornoy P, Bellaïche AEM, Merzoug V, Adamsbaum C. Fetal brain magnetic resonance imaging (MRI): indications, normal and pathological aspects. Revue neurologique 2009; 165(11):875-888.

45. Manganaro L, Bernardo S, De Vito C, Antonelli A, Marchionni E, Vinci V, et al. Role of fetal MRI in the evaluation of isolated and non-isolated corpus callosum dysgenesis: results of a cross-sectional study. Prenat Diagn. March 2017;37(3):244-52.

46. Rüland AM, Gloning K-P, Albig M, Kagan K-O, Hammer R, Schälike M, et al. The Incidence of Chromosomal Aberrations in Prenatally Diagnosed Isolated Agenesis of the Corpus Callosum. Ultraschall Med Stuttg Ger 1980. dec 2017;38(6):626-32.

47. Jeret JS, Serur D, Wisniewski KE, Lubin RA. Clinicopathological findings associated with agenesis of the corpus callosum. Brain Dev. 1987;9(3):255-64.

48. Shevell MI. Clinical and diagnostic profile of agenesis of the corpus callosum. J Child Neurol. Dec 2002;17(12):896-900.

49. Kim YU, Park ES, Jung S, Suh M, Choi HS, Rha D-W. Clinical features and associated abnormalities in children and adolescents with corpus callosal anomalies. Ann Rehabil Med. Feb 2014;38(1):138-43.

50 Goodyear PW, Bannister CM, Russell S, Rimmer S. Outcome in prenatally diagnosed fetal agenesis of the corpus callosum. Fetal Diagn Ther. June 2001;16(3):139-45.

51. Al-Hashim AH, Blaser S, Raybaud C, MacGregor D. Corpus callosum abnormalities: neuroradiological and clinical correlations. Dev Med Child Neurol. 2016;58(5):475-84.

52. Chen C-P, Lin S-P, Chang T-Y, Chiu N-C, Shih S-L, Lin C-J, et al. Perinatal imaging findings of inherited Sotos syndrome. Prenat Diagn. Oct 2002;22(10):887-92.

53. Gardiner K, Chitayat D, Choufani S, Shuman C, Blaser S, Terespolsky D, et al. Brain abnormalities in patients with Beckwith-Wiedemann syndrome. Am J Med Genet A. June 2012;158A(6):1388-94.

54. Jahani-Asl A, Cheng C, Zhang C, Bonni A. Pathogenesis of Börjeson-Forssman-Lehmann Syndrome: Insights from PHF6 Function. Neurobiol Dis. Dec 2016;96:227-35.

55. Szabó N, Gergev G, Kóbor J, Bereg E, Túri S, Sztriha L. Corpus callosum anomalies: birth prevalence and clinical spectrum in Hungary. Pediatr Neurol. June 2011;44(6):420-6.

56. Bedeschi MF, Bonaglia MC, Grasso R, Pellegri A, Garghentino RR, Battaglia MA, et al. Agenesis of the corpus callosum: clinical and genetic study in 63 young patients. Pediatr Neurol. March 2006;34(3):186-93.

57. Zhang W, Taylor SP, Ennis HA, Forlenza KN, Duran I, Li B, et al. Expanding the genetic architecture and phenotypic spectrum in the skeletal ciliopathies. Hum Mutat. 2018;39(1):152-66.

58. Laugel V. Cockayne syndrome: the expanding clinical and mutational spectrum. Mech Ageing Dev. June 2013;134(5-6):161-70.

59. Giraldo G, Gómez AM, Mora L, Suarez-Obando F, Moreno O. Mosaic trisomy 8 detected by fibroblasts cultured of skin. Colomb Médica CM. 47(2):100-4.

60. Margari L, Palumbi R, Campa MG, Operto FF, Buttiglione M, Craig F, et al. Clinical manifestations in children and adolescents with corpus callosum abnormalities. J Neurol. Oct 2016;263(10):1939-45.

61. Neal JB, Filippi CG, Mayeux R. Morphometric variability of neuroimaging features in children with agenesis of the corpus callosum. BMC Neurol. 25 Jul 2015;15:116.

62. Lábadi B, Beke AM. Mental State Understanding in Children with Agenesis of the Corpus Callosum. Front Psychol. 2017;8:94.

63. Paul LK, Corsello C, Kennedy DP, Adolphs R. Agenesis of the corpus callosum and autism: a comprehensive comparison. Brain J Neurol. June 2014;137(Pt 6):1813-29.

64. Volkmar F, Chawarska K, Klin A. Autism in infancy and early childhood. Annu Rev Psychol. 2005;56:315-36.

65. Badaruddin DH, Andrews GL, Bölte S, Schilmoeller KJ, Schilmoeller G, Paul LK, et al. Social and behavioral problems of children with agenesis of the corpus callosum. Child Psychiatry Hum Dev. Dec 2007;38(4):287-302.

66. Romaniello R, Arrigoni F, Bassi MT, Borgatti R. Mutations in α- and β-tubulin encoding genes: implications in brain malformations. Brain Dev. March 2015;37(3):273-80.

67. Welch KO, Tekin M, Nance WE, Blanton SH, Arnos KS, Pandya A. Chudley-McCullough syndrome: expanded phenotype and review of the literature. Am J Med Genet A. May 15, 2003;119A(1):71-6.

68. Chassaing N, Lacombe D, Carles D, Calvas P, Saura R, Bieth E. Donnai-Barrow syndrome: four additional patients. Am J Med Genet A. 1 Sep 2003;121A(3):258-62.

69. Hanna RM, Marsh SE, Swistun D, Al-Gazali L, Zaki MS, Abdel-Salam GM, et al. Distinguishing 3 classes of corpus callosal abnormalities in consanguineous families. Neurology. 25 Jan 2011;76(4):373-82.

70. Mordefroid M, Grabar S, André C, Merzoug V, Moutard M, Adamsbaum C. [Partial corpus callosum agenesis]. J Radiol. Nov 2004;85(11):1915-26.

71. Gelot A, Esperandieu O, Pompidou A. [Histogenesis of the corpus callosum]. Neurosurgery. May 1998;44(1 Suppl):61-73.

72. Knezović V, Kasprian G, Štajduhar A, Schwartz E, Weber M, Gruber GM, et al. Underdevelopment of the Human Hippocampus in Callosal Agenesis: An In Vivo Fetal MRI Study. AJNR Am J Neuroradiol. March 2019;40(3):576-81.

73. Zolotushko J, Flusser H, Markus B, Shelef I, Langer Y, Heverin M, et al. The desmosterolosis phenotype: spasticity, microcephaly and micrognathia with agenesis of corpus callosum and loss of white matter. Eur J Hum Genet EJHG. Sept 2011;19(9):942-6.

74. Lieb JM, Ahlhelm FJ. [Agenesis of the corpus callosum]. Radiol. Jul 2018;58(7):636-45.

75. O'Driscoll MC, Black GCM, Clayton-Smith J, Sherr EH, Dobyns WB. Identification of genomic loci contributing to agenesis of the corpus callosum. Am J Med Genet A. Sept 2010;152A(9):2145-59.

76. Chang Q, Zhong M, Yu Y, Xiong L, Chen C, Chen G, et al. [Prenatal diagnosis of agenesis of corpus callosum and its relationship with fetal chromosomal abnormalities]. Zhonghua Fu Chan Ke Za Zhi. nov 2013;48(11):810-4.

77. Heide S, Keren B, Billette de Villemeur T, Chantot-Bastaraud S, Depienne C, Nava C, et al. Copy Number Variations Found in Patients with a Corpus Callosum Abnormality and Intellectual Disability. J Pediatr. 2017;185:160-166.e1.

78. Mignot C, Moutard M-L, Rastetter A, Boutaud L, Heide S, Billette T, et al. ARID1B mutations are the major genetic cause of corpus callosum anomalies in patients with intellectual disability. Brain J Neurol. 01 2016;139(11):e64.

79. Edwards TJ, Sherr EH, Barkovich AJ, Richards LJ. Reply: ARID1B mutations are the major genetic cause of corpus callosum anomalies in patients with intellectual disability. Brain J Neurol. 01 2016;139(11):e65.

80. Thompson DK, Inder TE, Faggian N, Johnston L, Warfield SK, Anderson PJ, et al. Characterization of the corpus callosum in very preterm and full-term infants utilizing MRI. NeuroImage. March 15, 2011;55(2):479-90.

81. Prontera P, Bartocci A, Ottaviani V, Isidori I, Rogaia D, Ardisia C, et al. Aicardi Syndrome Associated with Autosomal Genomic Imbalance: Coincidence or Evidence for Autosomal Inheritance with Sex-Limited Expression? Mol Syndromol. 2013;4(4):197-202.

82. Govil-Dalela T, Kumar A, Agarwal R, Chugani HT. Agenesis of the Corpus Callosum and Aicardi Syndrome: A Neuroimaging and Clinical Comparison. Pediatr Neurol. 2017;68:44-48.e2.

83. Graham JM, Wheeler P, Tackels-Horne D, Lin AE, Hall BD, May M, et al. A new X-linked syndrome with agenesis of the corpus callosum, mental retardation, coloboma, micrognathia, and a mutation in the Alpha 4 gene at Xq13. Am J Med Genet A. 15 Nov 2003;123A(1):37-44.

84. Doherty D, Chudley AE, Coghlan G, Ishak GE, Innes AM, Lemire EG, et al. GPSM2 mutations cause the brain malformations and hearing loss in Chudley-McCullough syndrome. Am J Hum Genet. June 8, 2012;90(6):1088-93.

85. Ibisler A, Hehr U, Barth A, Koch M, Epplen JT, Hoffjan S. Novel KIF7 Mutation in a Tunisian Boy with Acrocallosal Syndrome: Case Report and Review of the Literature. Mol Syndromol. Oct 2015;6(4):173-80.

86. Putoux A, Baas D, Paschaki M, Morlé L, Maire C, Attié-Bitach T, et al. Altered GLI3 and FGF8 signaling underlies Acrocallosal syndrome phenotypes in Kif7 depleted mice. Hum Mol Genet. 15 Nov 2018;

87. Paetau A, Honkala H, Salonen R, Ignatius J, Kestilä M, Herva R. Hydrolethalus syndrome: neuropathology of 21 cases confirmed by HYLS1 gene mutation analysis. J Neuropathol Exp Neurol. August 2008;67(8):750-62.

88. Putoux A, Thomas S, Coene KLM, Davis EE, Alanay Y, Ogur G, et al. KIF7 mutations cause fetal hydrolethalus and acrocallosal syndromes. Nat Genet. June 2011;43(6):601-6.

89. Kato M, Das S, Petras K, Kitamura K, Morohashi K, Abuelo DN, et al. Mutations of ARX are associated with striking pleiotropy and consistent genotype-phenotype correlation. Hum Mutat. Feb 2004;23(2):147-59.

90. Jaglin XH, Poirier K, Saillour Y, Buhler E, Tian G, Bahi-Buisson N, et al. Mutations in the beta-tubulin gene TUBB2B result in asymmetrical polymicrogyria. Nat Genet. June 2009;41(6):746-52.

91. Howard HC, Dubé M-P, Prévost C, Bouchard J-P, Mathieu J, Rouleau GA. Fine mapping the candidate region for peripheral neuropathy with or without agenesis of the corpus callosum in the French Canadian population. Eur J Hum Genet EJHG. July 2002;10(7):406-12.

92. Bowerman M, Salsac C, Bernard V, Soulard C, Dionne A, Coque E, et al. KCC3 loss-of-function contributes to Andermann syndrome by inducing activity-dependent neuromuscular junction defects. Neurobiol Dis. Oct 2017;106:35-48.

93. Schaaf CP, Koster J, Katsonis P, Kratz L, Shchelochkov OA, Scaglia F, et al. Desmosterolosis-phenotypic and molecular characterization of a third case and review of the literature. Am J Med Genet A. Jul 2011;155A(7):1597-604.

94. Kortüm F, Jamra RA, Alawi M, Berry SA, Borck G, Helbig KL, et al. Clinical and genetic spectrum of AMPD2-related pontocerebellar hypoplasia type 9. Eur J Hum Genet EJHG. 2018;26(5):695-708.

95. Maillard C, Cavallin M, Piquand K, Philbert M, Bault JP, Millischer AE, et al. Prenatal and postnatal presentations of corpus callosum agenesis with polymicrogyria caused by EGP5 mutation. Am J Med Genet A. March 2017;173(3):706-11.

96. Khalifa O, Al-Sahlawi Z, Imtiaz F, Ramzan K, Allam R, Al-Mostafa A, et al. Variable expression pattern in Donnai-Barrow syndrome: Report of two novel LRP2 mutations and review of the literature. Eur J Med Genet. May 2015;58(5):293-9.

97. Koob M, Rousseau F, Laugel V, Meyer N, Armspach J-P, Girard N, et al. Cockayne syndrome: a diffusion tensor imaging and volumetric study. Br J Radiol. nov 2016;89(1067):20151033.

98. Wilson BT, Stark Z, Sutton RE, Danda S, Ekbote AV, Elsayed SM, et al. The Cockayne Syndrome Natural History (CoSyNH) study: clinical findings in 102 individuals and recommendations for care. Genet Med Off J Am Coll Med Genet. May 2016;18(5):483-93.

99. Bisschoff IJ, Zeschnigk C, Horn D, Wellek B, Rieß A, Wessels M, et al. Novel mutations including deletions of the entire OFD1 gene in 30 families with type I orofaciodigital syndrome: a study of the extensive clinical variability. Hum Mutat. Jan 2013;34(1):237-47.

100. Bruel A-L, Franco B, Duffourd Y, Thevenon J, Jego L, Lopez E, et al. Fifteen years of research on oral-facial-digital syndromes: from 1 to 16 causal genes. J Med Genet. 2017;54(6):371-80.

101. Poretti A, Snow J, Summers AC, Tekes A, Huisman TAGM, Aygun N, et al. Joubert syndrome: neuroimaging findings in 110 patients in correlation with cognitive function and genetic cause. J Med Genet. 2017;54(8):521-9.

102. Wang SF, Kowal TJ, Ning K, Koo EB, Wu AY, Mahajan VB, et al. Review of Ocular Manifestations of Joubert Syndrome. Genes (Basel). 2018 Dec 4;9(12).

103. Fleming LR, Doherty DA, Parisi MA, Glass IA, Bryant J, Fischer R, et al. Prospective Evaluation of Kidney Disease in Joubert Syndrome. Clin J Am Soc Nephrol CJASN. Dec 7, 2017;12(12):1962-73.

104. Karp N, Grosse-Wortmann L, Bowdin S. Severe aortic stenosis, bicuspid aortic valve and atrial septal defect in a child with Joubert Syndrome and Related Disorders (JSRD) -

a case report and review of congenital heart defects reported in the human ciliopathies. Eur J Med Genet. Nov 2012;55(11):605-10.

105. Bhoj EJ, Haye D, Toutain A, Bonneau D, Nielsen IK, Lund IB, et al. Phenotypic spectrum associated with SPECC1L pathogenic variants: new families and critical review of the nosology of Teebi, Opitz GBBB, and Baraitser-Winter syndromes. Eur J Med Genet. 22 Nov 2018;

106. Garavelli L, Ivanovski I, Caraffi SG, Santodirocco D, Pollazzon M, Cordelli DM, et al. Neuroimaging findings in Mowat-Wilson syndrome: a study of 54 patients. Genet Med Off J Am Coll Med Genet. 2017;19(6):691-700.

107. Ivanovski I, Djuric O, Caraffi SG, Santodirocco D, Pollazzon M, Rosato S, et al. Phenotype and genotype of 87 patients with Mowat-Wilson syndrome and recommendations for care. Genet Med Off J Am Coll Med Genet. 2018;20(9):965-75.

108. El-Hattab AW, Shaheen R, Hertecant J, Galadari HI, Albaqawi BS, Nabil A, et al. On the phenotypic spectrum of serine biosynthesis defects. J Inherit Metab Dis. 2016;39(3):373-81.

109. Darouich S, Boujelbene N, Kehila M, Chanoufi MB, Reziga H, Gaigi S, et al. [Neu-Laxova syndrome: Three case reports and a review of the literature]. Ann Pathol. August 2016;36(4):235-44.

110. Romaniello R, Arrigoni F, Fry AE, Bassi MT, Rees MI, Borgatti R, et al. Tubulin genes and malformations of cortical development. Eur J Med Genet. Dec 2018;61(12):744-54.

111. Birrell G, Lampe A, Richmond S, Bruce SN, Gécz J, Lower K, et al. Borjeson-Forssman-Lehmann syndrome and multiple pituitary hormone deficiency. J Pediatr Endocrinol Metab JPEM. Dec 2003;16(9):1295-300.

112. Shanske A, Caride DG, Menasse-Palmer L, Bogdanow A, Marion RW. Central nervous system anomalies in Seckel syndrome: report of a new family and review of the literature. Am J Med Genet. May 16, 1997;70(2):155-8.

113. Faivre L, Le Merrer M, Lyonnet S, Plauchu H, Dagoneau N, Campos-Xavier AB, et al. Clinical and genetic heterogeneity of Seckel syndrome. Am J Med Genet. 1 Nov 2002;112(4):379-83.

114. Verloes A, Drunat S, Gressens P, Passemard S. Primary Autosomal Recessive Microcephalies and Seckel Syndrome Spectrum Disorders. In: Adam MP, Ardinger HH, Pagon RA, Wallace SE, Bean LJ, Stephens K, et al., editors. GeneReviews®. Seattle (WA): University of Washington, Seattle; 1993-2019.

115. Magoulas PL, El-Hattab AW. Chromosome 15q24 microdeletion syndrome. Orphanet J Rare Dis. 4 Jan 2012;7:2.

116. Verstappen G, van Grunsven LA, Michiels C, Van de Putte T, Souopgui J, Van Damme J, et al. Atypical Mowat-Wilson patient confirms the importance of the novel

association between ZFHX1B/SIP1 and NuRD corepressor complex. Hum Mol Genet. 15 Apr 2008;17(8):1175-83.

117. Moldrich RX, Gobius I, Pollak T, Zhang J, Ren T, Brown L, et al. Molecular regulation of the developing commissural plate. J Comp Neurol. 15 Sep 2010;518(18):3645-61.

118. Douce JL. Metabolic alteration and synaptic deficit in Alzheimer's disease: role of astrocytic PHGDH.HAL open archives.dec 2015.

119. Grover VK, Valadez JG, Bowman AB, Cooper MK. Lipid modifications of Sonic hedgehog ligand dictate cellular reception and signal response. PloS One. 2011;6(7):e21353.

120. Moutard M-L, Kieffer V, Feingold J, Lewin F, Baron J-M, Adamsbaum C, et al. Isolated corpus callosum agenesis: a ten-year follow-up after prenatal diagnosis (how are the children without corpus callosum at 10 years of age?). Prenat Diagn. March 2012;32(3):277-83.

Appendices

APPENDICES

APPENDIX 1: Anatomy of the corpus callosum

The corpus callosum is the main inter-hemispheric commissure. It appears as a blade of transverse white matter that can be seen at the bottom of the interhemispheric fissure by moving the upper parts of the two cerebral hemispheres apart.

In medial sagittal section [Figure below], it appears C-shaped with a concavity at the bottom that corresponds posteriorly to the posterior edge of the cerebral trigone (fornix) and anteriorly to the septum pellucidum on the median line that separates the two lateral ventricles. Its convex upper surface is in line with the scythe of the brain, which insinuates itself into the inter-hemispheric scissure, and on the sides with the supra-callosal portion of the intra-limbic convolution.

It is made up of transversely arranged fibres and has several parts running from front to back, which connect the cerebral cortexes: the rostrum and knee unite the frontal cortexes, the body unites the parietal and temporal cortexes and the isthmus and splenium connect the occipital cortexes.

Vascularisation of the CC depends on the internal carotid system and the vertebro-basilar system.

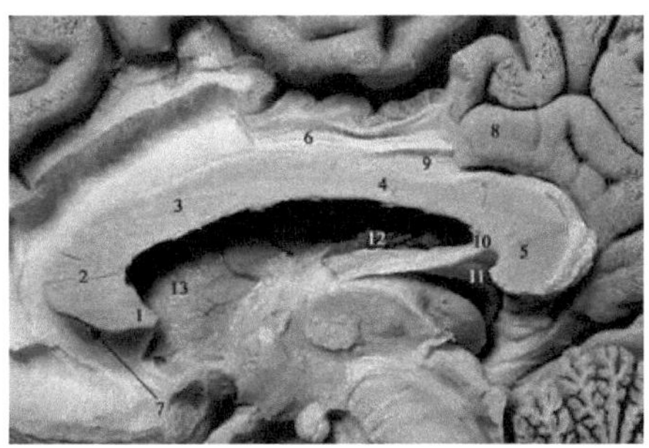

Sagittal medial section of the CC
(*Source: Anatomy of the human brain, Beal J., 2009*)

1: rostrum; 2: knee; 3: body; 4: isthmus; 5: splenium; 6: cingulate fibres; 7: subcallosal area; 8: cingulum; 9: indusium griseum; 10: calloso-forniceal adhesion; 11: crus fornicis; 12: choroid plexus; 13: head of caudate nucleus and right lateral ventricle.

APPENDIX 2: Clinical data collection form

Agenesis of the corpus callosum: Clinical form

<table>
<tr><td colspan="2">Patient no.: P</td><td>Family no.: F</td></tr>
<tr><td colspan="3">File number :</td></tr>
<tr><td colspan="3">Patient identity and family investigation</td></tr>
<tr><td colspan="2">Full name :</td><td></td></tr>
<tr><td colspan="2">Sex of patient :</td><td></td></tr>
<tr><td rowspan="2">Age</td><td>at the 1ère consultation:</td><td></td></tr>
<tr><td>at the last consultation :</td><td></td></tr>
<tr><td colspan="2">Addressing department :</td><td></td></tr>
<tr><td colspan="2">Reason for consultation :</td><td></td></tr>
<tr><td rowspan="2">Geographical origin</td><td>of the mother :</td><td></td></tr>
<tr><td>of the father :</td><td></td></tr>
<tr><td colspan="2">Parents' state of health :</td><td></td></tr>
<tr><td colspan="2">Consanguinity :</td><td>☐ NO
☐ YES</td></tr>
<tr><td rowspan="2">Family history</td><td>abnormality of the corpus callosum :</td><td>☐ NO
☐ YES Type :</td></tr>
<tr><td>other neurological impairment :</td><td>☐ NO
☐ YES Type :</td></tr>
<tr><td colspan="3">Pregnancy</td></tr>
<tr><td colspan="2">Mother's age at conception :</td><td></td></tr>
<tr><td rowspan="3">Special features of pregnancy</td><td>Design</td><td>☐ Spontaneous
☐ PMA</td></tr>
<tr><td>Morbidities in pregnancy :</td><td>☐ NO
☐ YES Type :</td></tr>
<tr><td>Taking medicines or toxic substances :</td><td>☐ NO
☐ YES Type :</td></tr>
<tr><td colspan="2">Pregnancy follow-up :</td><td>☐ NO
☐ YES</td></tr>
<tr><td colspan="2">Second trimester fetal ultrasound :</td><td>☐ NO
☐ YES Doctor specialising in foetal ultrasound: NO YES</td></tr>
<tr><td colspan="2">Prenatal ultrasound signs:</td><td>☐ NO
☐ YES Type :
Term :
Foetal MRI: NO YES</td></tr>
</table>

	Fetal MRI results :
Prenatal diagnosis :	☐ NO ☐ YES **Technical :** **Result:**
Birth	
Term	
Delivery route	
Biometrics at birth	**Weight = Height = PC =**
Personal history	
Tonus abnormalities :	☐ NO ☐ YES **Type :**
Eating disorders :	☐ NO ☐ YES
Engine delay :	☐ NO ☐ YES
Language delay :	☐ NO ☐ YES
Intellectual disability :	☐ NO ☐ YES **Degree :**
Epilepsy :	☐ NO ☐ YES **Type :**
Behavioural problems :	☐ NO ☐ YES **Type :**
Other special features:	
Clinical data	
Growth	**Height (DS) = Weight (DS) = (DS)** **Cranial perimeter (DS) = (in mm)**
Facial dysmorphia :	☐ NO ☐ YES **Details :** **Indicative of a particular syndrome**: NO YES
Extremity abnormalities :	☐ NO ☐ YES **Type :**
Other skeletal anomalies:	☐ NO ☐ YES **Type :**
Dermatoglyph anomalies :	☐ NO ☐ YES **Type :**
Skin and appendage abnormalities :	☐ NO ☐ YES **Type :**
OGE abnormalities :	☐ NO ☐ YES **Type :**

Abnormalities on cardiorespiratory examination		☐ NO ☐ YES **Type :**
Digestive abnormalities		☐ NO ☐ YES **Type :**
Ophthalmological abnormalities:		☐ NO ☐ YES **Type :**
Deafness		☐ NO ☐ YES
Neurological examination	**Toning**	
	Reflexes	
	Balance	
	Brain MRI data	
Type of ACC :		☐ Total ☐ Partial **agenesis segment:**
Indirect signs of ACC :		☐ Abnormalities of the lateral ventricles ☐ Anomalies of the 3rd ventricle ☐ Probst strips ☐ Circumvolution anomalies ☐ Abnormalities of other commissures **Description :**
Other malformations :		☐ Migration or gyration abnormalities ☐ White matter abnormalities ☐ Arachnoid cysts ☐ Inter-hemispheric cysts ☐ Abnormalities of the posterior fossa ☐ Eye abnormalities **Description :**
	Other investigations	
Cardiac ultrasound :		☐ NO ☐ YES **Result :**
Abdominal and pelvic imaging:		☐ NO ☐ YES **Result :**
Bone assessment :		☐ NO ☐ YES **Result :**
Metabolic balance :		☐ NO ☐ YES **Result :**
Other investigations :		☐ NO ☐ YES **Result :**
	Genetic study	
Karyotype :		
Other cytogenetic techniques		
Molecular biology :		

Diagnostic guidance	☐ NO ☐ YES **Diagnosis :**
PND subsequent pregnancy :	☐ NO ☐ YES

APPENDIX 3: The psychomotor development of infants and children.

Psychomotor development (PMD), linked to the maturation of the nervous system, concerns the child's motor and cognitive acquisitions and social interaction skills. The child's specific developmental process depends on genetic factors and factors interacting with the environment. The main stages in a child's MPD are summarised in the table below.

Age	Motor and postural acquisition	Grip	Acquisition language	Sensory acquisition Sociability	Cleanliness
2 months	Lift your head and shoulders	Grasping	Voice response to request	Smile answer	X
4 months	Headstand acquired	Grip on contact	Vocalise	Laughs out loud	X
6 months	Sits with support	Passes an object from one hand to the other	Babbling	Permanence de the object	X
9 months	- Sits without support - Stands with support	Thumb pliers-index	Repeat a syllable	- Fear of foreigners - Reacts to his first name	X
12-18 month	Walking alone	Stack 2 cubes	Match 2 words 7-10 words	- Understands simple sentences - Pointing objects	X
24 months	Short	Copy a line	First phrases	Wash and dry your hands	Cleanliness diurnal
3 years	Climb the stairs alternately	Copy a circle, a cross	Tells a little story	Autonomy for undressing	Cleanliness night

Psychomotor delay is defined as the failure to acquire developmental norms at the programmed ages. A psychomotor delay may be global (affecting all types of acquisition), or concern only one of them. In terms of postural acquisition, delayed acquisition is defined as the absence of sitting up by 9 months and the absence of independent walking by 18 months. Delayed language acquisition is defined by an absence of canonical babbling at 9 months, an absence of words at 15 months and an absence of sentences at 3 years.

APPENDIX 4: Example of Phenomizer search results

Phenomizer Diagnosis Report April 1, 2019

1 Patient data

Name, Firstname: P19

Date of birth:

Gender: Male ★ Female

2 Query

Query Terms:

- Delayed ossification of carpal bones (HP:0001216)
- Camptodactyly (HP:0012385)
- Myopia (HP:0000545)
- Intellectual disability (HP:0001249)
- Intrauterine growth retardation (HP:0001511)
- Joint laxity (HP:0001388)
- Hearing impairment (HP:0000365)
- Global developmental delay (HP:0001263)
- Partial agenesis of the corpus callosum (HP:0001338)
- Abnormal localization of kidney (HP:0100542)

Inheritance: none

Similarity measure: Resnik (not symmetric)

3 Results

p-Value	*Score*	*Disease entry*	*Known Genes*
0.0160	2.2809	#614815 JOUBERT SYNDROME 18; JBTS18 (OMIM:614815)	OFD1, C5ORF42, TCTN3, TMEM216, KIF7, PDE6D
0.1602	1.6438	15Q24 RECURRENT MICRODELETION SYNDROME (DECIPHER:66)	

Reference:
Köhler S, Schulz MH, Krawitz P, Bauer S, Dölken S, Ott CE, Mundlos C, Horn D, Mundlos S, Robinson PN
Clinical Diagnostics in Human Genetics with Semantic Similarity Searches in Ontologies
The American Journal of Human Genetics 85, pp. 457-464, Oktober 2009.

p-Value	*Score*	*Disease entry*	*Known Genes*
0.2624	2.2185	#120330 PAPILLORENAL SYNDROME; PAPRS;;RENAL-COLOBOMA SYNDROME;;OPTIC NERVE COLOBOMA WITH RENAL DISEASE;;COLOBOMA OF OPTIC NERVE WITH RENAL DISEASE;;OPTIC COLOBOMA, VESICOURETERAL REFLUX, AND RENAL ANOMALIES;;RENAL-COLOBOMA SYNDROME WITH MACULAR ABNORMALITIES;;CONGENITAL ANOMALIES OF THE KIDNEY AND URINARY TRACT WITH OCULAR ABNORMALITIES;;CAKUT WITH OCULAR ABNORMALITIES (OMIM:120330)	PAX2
0.2624	2.0460	#614851 SECKEL SYNDROME 7; SCKL7 (OMIM:614851)	NIN
0.2624	1.7505	#616081 PONTOCEREBELLAR HYPOPLASIA, TYPE 1C; PCH1C;;HYPOMYELINATION WITH SPINAL MUSCULAR ATROPHY AND CEREBELLAR HYPOPLASIA (OMIM:616081)	TSEN54, EXOSC3, VRK1, EXOSC8, RARS2
0.2624	1.6844	%217990 CORPUS CALLOSUM, AGENESIS OF;;ACC (OMIM:217990)	
0.2624	1.6265	#613162 SPASTIC PARAPLEGIA 45, AUTOSOMAL RECESSIVE; SPG45 (OMIM:613162)	NT5C2
0.2624	1.6036	#615282 CORTICAL DYSPLASIA, COMPLEX, WITH OTHER BRAIN MALFORMATIONS 2; CDCBM2 (OMIM:615282)	KIF5C
0.2624	1.4548	#615807 SECKEL SYNDROME 8; SCKL8 (OMIM:615807)	ATR, DNA2, CEP152, CENPE, CENPJ, PCNT, RBBP8, PLK4, ATRIP
0.2624	1.4040	#615411 CORTICAL DYSPLASIA, COMPLEX, WITH OTHER BRAIN MALFORMATIONS 3; CDCBM3 (OMIM:615411)	KIF2A

4 Further analysis

(Shown is a list of features that are special to the corresponding OMIM entry and not shared by another OMIM entry from the result list.)

OMIM entry	*Features*
#614815 JOUBERT SYNDROME 18; JBTS18 (OMIM:614815)	

Reference:

Köhler S, Schulz MH, Krawitz P, Bauer S, Dölken S, Ott CE, Mundlos C, Horn D, Mundlos S, Robinson PN
Clinical Diagnostics in Human Genetics with Semantic Similarity Searches in Ontologies
The American Journal of Human Genetics 85, pp. 457-464, Oktober 2009.

OMIM entry	*Features*
15Q24 RECURRENT MICRODELETION SYNDROME (DECIPHER:66)	
#120330 PAPILLORENAL SYNDROME; PAPRS;;RENAL-COLOBOMA SYNDROME;;OPTIC NERVE COLOBOMA WITH RENAL DISEASE;;COLOBOMA OF OPTIC NERVE WITH RENAL DISEASE;;OPTIC COLOBOMA, VESICOURETERAL REFLUX, AND RENAL ANOMALIES;;RENAL-COLOBOMA SYNDROME WITH MACULAR ABNORMALITIES;;CONGENITAL ANOMALIES OF THE KIDNEY AND URINARY TRACT WITH OCULAR ABNORMALITIES;;CAKUT WITH OCULAR ABNORMALITIES (OMIM:120330)	
#614851 SECKEL SYNDROME 7; SCKL7 (OMIM:614851)	
#616081 PONTOCEREBELLAR HYPOPLASIA, TYPE 1C; PCH1C;;HYPOMYELINATION WITH SPINAL MUSCULAR ATROPHY AND CEREBELLAR HYPOPLASIA (OMIM:616081)	
%217990 CORPUS CALLOSUM, AGENESIS OF;;ACC (OMIM:217990)	
#613162 SPASTIC PARAPLEGIA 45, AUTOSOMAL RECESSIVE; SPG45 (OMIM:613162)	
#615282 CORTICAL DYSPLASIA, COMPLEX, WITH OTHER BRAIN MALFORMATIONS 2; CDCBM2 (OMIM:615282)	
#615807 SECKEL SYNDROME 8; SCKL8 (OMIM:615807)	
#615411 CORTICAL DYSPLASIA, COMPLEX, WITH OTHER BRAIN MALFORMATIONS 3; CDCBM3 (OMIM:615411)	**Abnormality of the nervous system:** - Pachygyria (HP:0001302) - Lissencephaly (HP:0001339)

Reference:
Köhler S, Schulz MH, Krawitz P, Bauer S, Dölken S, Ott CE, Mundlos C, Horn D, Mundlos S, Robinson PN
Clinical Diagnostics in Human Genetics with Semantic Similarity Searches in Ontologies
The American Journal of Human Genetics 85, pp. 457-464, Oktober 2009.

APPENDIX 5: Consent form for patients' legal representatives

TUNISIAN REPUBLIC
MINISTRY OF HEALTH
DISEASE CONTROL
CONGENITAL AND HEREDITARY
Head of Department: Pr M'RAD Ridha

Consent form for a genetic study

I, the undersigned :
Surname: First name: born on :

Acting as the patient's parent/legal representative :
Surname: First name: born on :

Certify that I have been fully informed by Doctor :
Last name: First name :

Address:

1- The reasons for and conditions of the genetic study concerning me/my minor child
2- The help that genetic tests can provide in diagnosing the disease and, where appropriate, preventing it or treating its complications
3- The strictly confidential nature of the results obtained
4- That my attending physician will be able to inform me of the results and of any confidential information concerning me/my minor child
5- That these studies will be carried out by a specialised, accredited laboratory
6- That I could ask for the study to be stopped at any time and for the samples to be returned to me.

- **Authorises a direct debit to be taken from** :
  - Myself
  - My child

For the purpose of investigating the origin of the medical problem for which I have been referred to this doctor, by studying the DNA using molecular biology or molecular cytogenetic techniques and/or by examining the chromosomes.

- **Agrees that the samples taken may be used for these** examinations

- **I agree to the collection, processing and recording of the data contained in the medical file required for these studies.**

Signed in Tunis on
Signature of the person concerned

Name and signature of prescribing doctor

Signature of parent/legal guardian

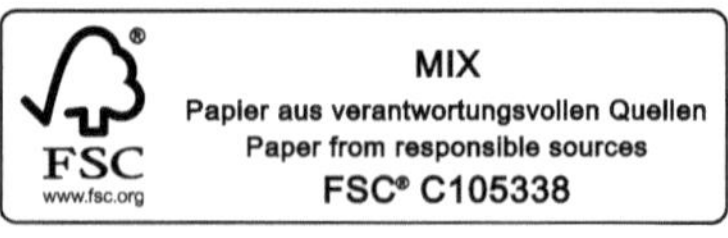

Printed by Books on Demand GmbH, Norderstedt / Germany